MEDICINE FOR WOMEN
IN IMPERIAL CHINA

MEDICINE FOR WOMEN IN IMPERIAL CHINA

EDITED BY

ANGELA KI CHE LEUNG

BRILL
LEIDEN • BOSTON
2006

The content of this volume is a reprint
of volume 7, issue 2 (2005) of
*Nan Nü, Men, Women
and Gender in China.*

ISBN 90 04 15196 6

Brill
Leiden · Boston

ISSN 0022-4995

CONTENTS

FOREWORD

This issue of *NAN NÜ*, focused on medicine for women in imperial China, is the third special theme number to appear since the journal's founding seven years ago. Like the earlier theme issues, one on female suicide (3.1 [2001]) and the other on gender and genre in late Qing China (6.1 [2004]), this number will be published as a separate book volume. But unlike these two previous numbers, this issue did not originate from an earlier academic meeting or panel presentation. For the last several years, Angela Leung, the special guest editor of this issue, and I had been discussing the possibility of organizing a *NAN NÜ* issue which would highlight some of the more recent trends in the study of Chinese medicine for women. With the publication of the path-breaking book by Charlotte Furth, *A Flourishing Yin: Gender in China's Medical History, 960-1665* (Berkeley: University of California Press, 1999), this particular specialization within the discipline of the history of Chinese medicine is now attracting ever more interest, both in East Asia and in Euro-America. We are pleased that a group of distinguished scholars, including Professor Furth herself, agreed to contribute their expertise to this theme issue. It is this kind of joint effort which helps make the study of men, women and gender in China such a dynamic and exciting field of research and analysis. And the *NAN NÜ* Board of Editors hopes to continue publishing on special themes in the future, to keep both China scholars and the broader public alert to further developments in gender study.

Harriet T. Zurndorfer

RECENT TRENDS IN THE STUDY OF MEDICINE FOR WOMEN IN IMPERIAL CHINA

BY

ANGELA KI CHE LEUNG
(Institute of History and Philology, Academia Sinica)

Strictly speaking, women and medicine in Chinese history is not an entirely new field. Historians of Chinese medicine trained during the first half of the twentieth century such as Xie Guan 謝觀 (1880-1950), Fan Xingzhun 范行準 (1906-98), and Zhao Pushan 趙璞珊 (1926-), who had great influence on subsequent generations of historians of medicine in China, already traced the development of "medicine for women" in their classic works on the general history of Chinese medicine.[1] Both Fan and Xie described the development of medicine for women in the Sui-Tang period, and Xie, in particular, provided a short, clear, and typically insightful historical development of what he called *nüke xue* 女科學 (learning on medicine for women), from Tang dynasty Zan Yin 昝殷 (ninth century) to Qing experts, quoting major works and their characteristics. Zhao Pushan, a specialist in the history of Chinese pediatrics and Song-Yuan medicine also substantially quotes Tang works on obstetrics and points out pertinently that the landmark innovation of Song works on *fuke* 婦科 (gynecology) was the emphasis on the regulation of menses.[2] Another important Chinese historian of medicine, Li Jingwei 李經緯 (1929-), more

---

[1] Xie Liheng 謝利恆 (Xie Guan 謝觀), *Zhongguo yixue yuanliu lun* 中國醫學源流論 (Taibei: Guting shudian, 1970); Fan Xingzhun, *Zhongguo yixue shilue* 中國醫學史略 (Beijing: Zhongyi guji chubanshe, 1986); his *Zhongguo bingshi xinyi* 中國病史新義 (Beijing: Zhongguo guji chubanshe, 1989) provides ample early examples of discussions of disorders specific to women in both medical and nonmedical texts; see pp. 560-82; Zhao Pushan, *Zhongguo gudai yixue* 中國古代醫學 (1983; reprint, Beijing: Zhonghua shuju, 1997); Li Jingwei 李經緯 and Li Zhidong 李志東, *Zhongguo gudai yixue shilue* 中國古代醫學史略 (Shijiazhuang: Heibei kexue jishu chubanshe, 1990), 187-90.

[2] Xie Liheng, *Zhongguo yixue yuanliu lun*, 38-39; Zhao Pushan, *Zhongguo gudai yixue*, 132-34.

Also available online – www.brill.nl

recently gives further weight to the importance of *fuke* development in the Song by providing a detailed account of the representative *fuke* expert, Chen Ziming 陳自明 (ca. 1190-1270). In the 1980s a second generation of historians indicated clearly that by Song times, *fuke* was separated from internal medicine and became a separate discipline.[3] This interest in the development of *fuke* within the framework of the general history of medicine in China paved the way for the publication in 1991 of Ma Dazheng's 馬大正 book on the specific history of Chinese gynecology.[4] Historians like Zhang Zhibin 張志斌, who published her work on gynecological disorders in 2000, discussed by Ricardo Mak in this issue, represent the third generation of Chinese historians of medicine for women.[5] All of these works come from the modern tradition of Chinese medical history beginning in the early twentieth century, with only marginal interest in the social or cultural background of such history.

The feminist or cultural approaches to the history of *fuke*, and to a broader narrative of women, body, and medicine in history, on the other hand, is a new development that becomes visible only from the late 1990s onwards. Major publications in this field come mainly from America and Taiwan. The present *Nan Nü* issue clearly shows this trend. A major landmark in this recent and exciting development is obviously Charlotte Furth's groundbreaking work: *A Flourishing Yin: Gender in China's Medical History, 960-1665* (Berkeley: University of California Press, 1999). Readers will find that two of the three major articles in this issue (those by Yates and Wilms) are inspired by this book, whereas Lee Jen-der's 李貞德 article, translated from its 1996 Chinese version, is one of Furth's reference works. These three articles treat historical developments prior to Furth's main period of interest. This is interesting because they all address a significant point made by earlier works by Chinese historians of medicine as well as by Furth: the maturation of Chinese *fuke* during the Song. The obvious question they all try to answer is the following: what paved the way to Song *fuke*? Could one in fact talk about the first

---

[3] Anonymous, *Zhongguo yiyao shihua* 中國醫藥史話 (Taibei: Mingwen shuju, 1983), 248-49.

[4] Ma Dazheng , *Zhongguo fuchanke fazhan shi* 中國婦產科發展史 (Xi'an: Shaanxi kexue jiaoyu chubanshe, 1991).

[5] Zhang Zhibin, *Gudai zhongyi fuchanke jibing shi* 古代中醫婦產科疾病史 (Beijing: Zhongyi guji chubanshe, 2000).

formulation of a coherent body of learning on medicine for women already in the Tang period, as Xie Guan had already done?

The Significance of Furth's "A Flourishing Yin"

Furth's book has clearly made its impact on both the study of the Chinese history of medicine and in the cultural analysis of the history of the body, and its influence will certainly expand if it is translated into Asian languages, especially Chinese. Furth's purpose in writing this book is threefold: to write a history of medicine, to address the question of gender in medicine, and to make a discourse analysis relating woman's medical body to her social body. In other words, this book is at the same time a sinological description of *fuke* as a medical discipline meaningful to traditional historians of Chinese medicine and an analysis of *fuke*, or the female body as a construct based on words and language in a specific cultural context, a fruitful approach already taken by many Western feminist scholars, notably Thomas Laqueur and Barbara Duden, whose works inspired Furth.[6] Furth's book has admirably achieved the difficult goals that the author set for herself, and it is a rich history of *fuke* not only as a medical practice and a cultural construct, but also as an intelligible social exercise carried out by relevant actors—men, women, scholars, male doctors, midwives, female healers, and so on—and a body of thought closely articulating with the development of Neo-Confucianism since the Song. This book is a carefully constructed social history with a sophisticated theoretical framework.

The main arguments of the book build around the tension between the ideal and ahistorical androgynous body that Furth named "the Yellow Emperor's body," and the female gestational body that clearly distinguished itself in the Song. While Furth bases her analysis of the androgynous body mainly on the late imperial interpretations of the medical classic, the *Inner Canon*, Lisa Raphals has reached a similar

---

[6] Furth admits in the introduction (p. 4) that her book was inspired by works by these two scholars and by Roy Porter ed., *Patients and Practitioners: Lay Perception of Medicine in Pre-Industrial Societies*. (Cambridge: Cambridge University Press, 1985). In terms of discourse analysis, the works of Duden and Laqueur seem to have greater influence on this book. See Barbara Duden, *The Woman Beneath the Skin: A Doctor's Patients in Eighteenth-century Germany* (Cambridge, Mass.: Harvard University Press, 1991); Thomas Laqueur, *Making Sex: Body and Gender from the Greeks to Freud* (Cambridge, Mass.: Harvard University Press, 1990).

conclusion by studying the cases of the early doctor Chunyu Yi 淳于意 (third century BC) described in the *Shiji* 史記—that there was a lack of emphasis on sexual difference in his medical diagnoses.[7] Furth's inspiration, however, seems to have come essentially from Laqueur, although one must be cautious not to confuse her arguments with Laqueur's viewpoints. While Laqueur eloquently discusses the "one-sex" body conceptualized by the Ancient Greeks and lasting through the Renaissance, giving way to the well-bounded, gendered "two-sex" bodies after the eighteenth century, Furth's Yellow Emperor's body was androgynous but not "one-sex," and the development of the female gestational body was not linear like that of the well-gendered body in the modern West. The androgynous body, a generative body containing both *yin* and *yang*, was an ideal body in which sex was not the focus of attention, especially towards the later imperial period. The female gestational body of Song *fuke*, characterized by "Blood as the leader" as distinct from the male-based androgynous body, on the other hand, retreated after the Ming. For Furth, Ming and Qing *fuke* specialists stepped back from the Song thesis of "Blood as the leader" characterizing the female body, and, contrary to their Song predecessors, interpreted many female disorders as non-gender-specific. *Fuke* shrank from concerns of a more general, holistic female body to increasingly specific gestational problems. The ideal of the androgynous body had returned forcefully under the influence of Ming-Qing Neo-Confucianism. The *yin/yang* balance of the viscera, common to bodies of both sexes and reflecting the intellectual and mental well-being of a person, became an increasingly important measure of health compared with a decreasing emphasis on unique "Blood" for appraising the various pathological problems of the female body. "Flourishing *yin*" (*jiyin* 濟陰) became a late imperial model remedy for a body typically overwhelmed with *yang*, that is, saturated with excessive desires and mundane activities, a problem that preoccupied Neo-Confucian doctors. Joanna Grant's *A Chinese Physician: Wang Ji and the "Stone Mountain Medical Case Histories"* (2003), finely reviewed by Marta Hanson in this issue, shows some of such changes in the late imperial period through the clinical experience of the Ming doctor Wang Ji 汪機 (1463-1539).

In fact, the careful reader could make interesting contrasts between

---

[7] Lisa Raphals, "The Treatment of Women in a Second-century Medical Casebook," *Chinese Science* 15 (1998): 7-23.

Furth's and Laqueur's books. While most discussions and descriptions in *A Flourishing Yin* are on the gestational problems of the female body, *Making Sex* is more on the anatomy of the genitalia and sex itself. Indeed, the question of female orgasm and its relation to conception ran through the entire book. While Furth's book clearly captures one increasingly central concern of post-Song Chinese society, the production of male heirs for ancestor worship, Laqueur's discussions reveal the obsession with sex in Western religion and medicine. In China, the technique of prolonged sexual combat and "plucking *yin* to replenish *yang*" by rousing female orgasm, central in the Sui-Tang Daoist bodily technique of "nourishing life" for elite males, fell out of fashion in late imperial *yangsheng* 養生 discourse.[8] Self-cultivation of Essence, focusing Psyche, and sexual moderation now became the key to the male fertile body central to the perpetuation of the family line in the Ming-Qing period. Indeed, contrary to the modern West, Chinese society viewed sex as increasingly secondary to and inseparable from reproduction.

The richness of Furth's discussions and the originality of her arguments will certainly inspire related works to come in the near future, both in medical history and in gender studies. As clearly shown in the title of her book, the main discussions in the book are on the later imperial period beginning from the Song. Though Furth provides information on developments in medicine for women prior to the Song, the descriptions are necessarily brief. The present issue shows that in the history of medicine, there is still much room for further research on the periods before the tenth century.

Early Medicine for Women

The three rich sinological studies in this issue on women, childbirth, and medicine in China from antiquity to the Sui-Tang periods constitute a coherent ensemble nicely complementing Furth's work on the later imperial periods. Even though none of the three papers takes the discourse analysis approach that marks Furth's work, they are useful in revealing the rich and complex tradition that Song *fuke* specialists had inherited. In many ways, they show how the guiding theme of Song gynecology highlighted by Furth, "Blood is the leader," had been constructed during the preceding periods.

---

[8] Furth, *A Flourishing Yin*, 202.

Robin Yates's paper, "Medicine for Women in Early China: A Preliminary Survey," particularly informative on ancient texts and archaeological findings, provides a complex picture of the formative period of medicine for women and argues that medicine was clearly gendered in the Sui-Tang period. While reminding us of the frustrating loss of many early relevant texts that might contain important information, it pertinently highlights the omnipresence of religious and ritual elements in early medicine, right down to the Sui-Tang period, an indicator of the importance of the Buddhist and Daoist traditions. The author is particularly sensitive to the issues of pollution, taboos, and related rituals: the discussions on the *yin* nature of toilets, the use of cloth as an ingredient in concoctions for terminating pregnancies, food proscriptions for pregnant women, and incantations during delivery, for instance, contain many insightful remarks. Discussions of little-explored medicinal treatments related to the female body, such as fragrances, unguents to counter aging, and care of the hair, for instance, remind the reader of the importance of physiognomy in early China. This paper rightly emphasizes the complex meaning of what could be framed as "medicine" for women in early China and its heavy religious content, which gradually diminished after the Song.

Wilms's paper, "'Ten Times More Difficult to Treat': Female Bodies in Medical Texts from Early Imperial China," on the other hand, is focused on pathological problems based on early mainstream medical classics. Its main ideas are clearly inspired by Furth's book, and the article is a useful complementary reading. It directly addresses one of Furth's main arguments, that Song *fuke* is distinct by claiming "Blood as the leader" in the female body, explaining how this notion was gradually constructed during the earlier periods. The author traces the gendering of medicine from the Han to the Song period by scrutinizing the question of female pathology directly related to gestation and childbirth, summarized as a broad category of "below the girdle" (*daixia* 帶下) in early China. While vaginal discharges were a main concern for Sui-Tang doctors such as Chao Yuanfang 巢元方 (early seventh century), Sun Simiao 孫思邈 (ca 581-682), several decades later, stressed the problem of "noxious dew" (*e lu* 惡露; old Blood left over in the womb after childbirth). Wilms argues that though Sun described the distinctiveness of the female body with Blood as the source of most of its pathological problems, he spoke more like a hands-on "technician" and did not theorize about the problem. The theoretical construct of a gendered and holistic female body based on "Blood as the leader" was achieved by experts only in the Song, notably by Chen Ziming. On this Wilms entirely agrees with Furth on the significance and characteristics of the development of Song *fuke*.

Lee Jen-der's "Childbirth in Early Imperial China" was published in Chinese in 1996 and quoted in Furth's book together with her other paper, "Han-Tang zhijian qiuzi yifang shitan—jianlun fuke lanshang yu xingbie lunshu" 漢唐之間求子醫方試探—兼論婦科濫觴與性別論述, published in 1997.[9] In the latter, Lee argues that the beginning of a coherent corpus of medical knowledge about the specific female body was emerging in the Tang. The paper in this issue deals more specifically with childbirth as a central problem of the female body, including preparation for the birth, the delivery process, and postpartum problems as a medical as well as a social concern. This paper reveals the rich and complex tradition surrounding childbirth from the Qin to the Tang periods, built not only upon technical obstetric advice but also on ritual practices, particularly in regard to the problem of pollution related to Blood. Both medical and religious considerations constituted an inseparable body of knowledge that Song *fuke* experts had inherited. With concrete examples from medical and various nonmedical primary sources, Lee shows how anxieties in regard to childbirth in the early period helped to construct an elaborate and coherent body of medical and ritual techniques known as *fuke* that formed the basis for the later development of medicine for women.

These three authors in this issue stress the important contribution of Tang doctors, especially Sun Simiao, in the construct of *fuke*. They note in slightly different ways that the female body acquired new importance in mainstream medicine during this period. Yates clearly thinks that the gendering of body and medicine began in Tang texts, while Wilms admits the innovation of Sun Simiao in focusing on the distinct characteristics of the female body necessitating special medical care, though the gendered body was fully conceptualized only in the Song. Lee does not directly address the question of body gendering in her article here but discusses the question in her 1997 article, where she stresses that it was during the Tang that the medical discourse

[9] Lee Jen-der, "Han-Tang zhijian qiuzi yifang shitan jianlun fuke lanshang yu xingbie lunshu", *Bulletin of the Institute of History and Philology, Academia Sinica* 中央研究院歷史語言研究所集刊 68.2 (1997): 283-367.

recognizing the specificity of the female body emerged. She quotes at length the passage "*furen fang*" 婦人方 (prescriptions for women) in Sun Simiao's text to show that it "established the notion of gender differences announcing the beginning of *fuke* medicine."[10] A key question is therefore whether Song *fuke* was truly a different paradigm from the "early *fuke*" in the Tang,[11] a central theme in Furth's book. For Furth, one main indicator of the conceptualization of the female body as a gendered and holistic entity is that the old category of *daixia*, an umbrella covering broad groups of miscellaneous disorders (*zabing* 雜病) of the female body, was still maintained in Tang medical texts and was reduced to a specific diagnostic category of leukorrhea only in the Song. Indeed, she thinks that only when female *zabing* not necessarily related to gestation were discussed as an inherent part of *fuke,* as they were in the Song, can we consider medicine fully gendered. By looking at the shrinking *zabing* category in Ming *fuke,* Furth concludes that the gendering of medicine went "backwards" in the late imperial period when many of these disorders were reclassified as ungendered ones related to the androgynous body.[12] Because the main focus of these three authors in this issue is on childbirth and female gestational problems and not the other pathological problems of women, no full debate is engaged with Furth on the question of the definition and periodization of the gendering of medicine in China, even though all agree that more attention should be paid to the development of medicine for women in the earlier periods.[13] In fact, Li Jianmin 李建民 has more recently proposed another angle from which to consider the conceptualization of a gendered body in early China. He suggests that the male body was conceptualized around the functions of the *dumai* 督脈 (superintendent channel, or central vessel) as described in the *Inner Canon*, especially its role in the early art of "nourishing life."[14] While it is still unclear how Li's point will engage with Furth's idea of the androgynous body, one

[10] Lee, "Han-Tang zhijian qiuzi," 316.

[11] This is the term used by Furth, *A Flourishing Yin,* 64.

[12] Furth, *A Flourishing Yin,* 166-68.

[13] Another argument proposed by Furth on the question of gendering is based on the bodily technique of "nourishing life" by inner alchemy, *neidan* 內丹, analyzed in Ch. 6.

[14] Li Jianmin, "Dumai yu Zhongguo zaoqi yangsheng shijian: qi jing ba mai di xin yanjiu zhi er" 督脈與中國早期養生實踐：奇經八脈的新研究之二, *Bulletin of the Institute of History and Philology, Academia Sinica* 76.2 (2005):249-314.

can certainly look forward to more lively and constructive discussions on the issue in the near future.

Other Recent Works on Medicine and Women

Medicine for women in imperial China as a new area of interest is certainly growing. The main scholars in the field are no doubt Furth, specializing in the late imperial period, and Lee, expert on early China to the Sui-Tang periods. Since 1995, Lee has published nine sinological articles in Chinese on medicine and women in the early period, of which two, including the present one, have been translated into English and published in this journal.[15] In these articles Lee systematically treats two main aspects of women, health, and medicine from early China to the Sui-Tang periods: the role of women as caretakers of health and the female gestational body. Her approach is both medical and social, and many of her conclusions evoke the interesting observation made by Furth that Chinese "bodily gender was a plastic androgyny while social gender was based on fixed hierarchy."[16] For instance, while parts of the female body could be used as ingredients in drugs in the pharmacopeia, the presence of women was forbidden in the drug-making process because the female body was considered to be naturally polluting and taboo.

---

[15] Besides her article in this issue, the above-mentioned 1997 article quoted by Furth (See note 9) , and her other paper published in this journal, "Wet Nurses in Early Imperial China," *Nan Nü* 2.1 (2000):1-39 (translated from "Han-Wei Liuchao di rumu" 漢魏六朝的乳母, *Bulletin of the Institute of History and Philology, Academia Sinica* 70.2 (1999):439-81, her other papers are: 1) "Han-Sui zhijian di shengzi buju wenti" 漢隋之間的生子不舉問題，*Bulletin of the Institute of History and Philology, Academia Sinica* 66.3 (1995):747-812; 2) "Han-Tang zhijian di nüxing yiliao zhaogu zhe" 漢唐之間的女性醫療照顧者,*Taida lishi xuebao* 台大歷史學報23 (1999):123-56; 3) "Han-Tang zhijian yifang zhong di ji jian furen yu nüti wei yao" 漢唐之間醫方中的忌見婦人與女體爲藥, *Xinshixue* 新史學 (Taipei), 13.4 (2002):1-36; 4) "Han-Tang zhijian jiating zhong di jiankang zhaogu yu xingbie" 漢唐之間家庭中的健康照顧與性別 in *Gender and Medical History: Papers From the Third International Conference on Sinology, History Section* 第三屆國際漢學會議論文集－性別與醫療- 歷史組, edited by K. W. Huang 黃克武, (Academia Sinica: Institute of Modern History (2003), 1-50; 5) "Tangdai di xingbie yu yiliao" 唐代的性別與醫療, *Tang-Song nüxing yu shehui* 唐宋女性與社會, in Deng Xiaonan 鄧小南, ed. (Shanghai: Shanghai Cishu chubanshe, 2003), 415-46; 6) " '*Ishinpo'* lun 'furen zhubing suoyou' ji qi xiangguan wenti" (『醫心方』論「婦人諸病所由」及其相關問題), *Tsing Hua Journal of Chinese Studies* 清華學報 34.2 (2004): 479-511.

[16] Furth, *A Flourishing Yin*, 305.

When the responsibility of conception was shifting from men to women as suggested in medical texts of the Sui-Tang period, male doctors dominated the discourse on the female gestational body and tended to intervene more directly in childbirth even though many of them were inexperienced technicians in this domain. Female healers, midwives, wet nurses, neighbors, and relatives, on the other hand, continued to play significant roles inside and outside the family as helpers in childbirth, under the suspicious eye of the male doctor. The feminist position of Lee is not arrived at by discourse analysis as in Furth's case, but by meticulous scrutiny of all kinds of early texts that show the predicament of early female health caretakers to be not so different from that of today: daughters, wives, and mothers were considered "natural" caretakers of health who often find themselves in conflicting situations in the "inner sphere," whereas sons' and husbands' caretaking responsibility rarely provoked conflicts and was often publicized as virtue that could enhance their public image or career. The well-defined social limits and obligations imposed on female (and male) healers and health caretakers contrast interestingly with the vulnerable and polluting nature of the female body, whose generative role was portrayed by medical texts as an ungraspable problem. Indeed, Lee shows us with numerous concrete examples that while the gendered social hierarchy was stable and fixed, the boundaries of the gendered body were fluid, changeable, and problematic.

The ungraspable nature of the female gestational body continued to preoccupy medical authors well into the late imperial period, as finely analyzed in Yi-li Wu's 2002 article published in this journal, "Ghost Fetuses, False Pregnancies, and the Parameters of Medical Uncertainty in Classical Chinese Gynecology."[17] Wu, whose research on Qing *fuke* will soon appear in the form of a book,[18] is another scholar who has made important contributions to the field of medicine and women in recent years. Specialized in Ming-Qing medicine for women, Wu has enriched our understanding of the female body as described in late imperial medical texts by focusing on its specific

[17] *Nan Nü* 4.2 (2002):170-206.

[18] Her article in *Late Imperial China* 21.1 (2000):41-76, "The Bamboo Grove Monastery and Popular Gynecology in Qing China," reveals some emphases of her 1992 Ph.D. dissertation: "Transmitted Secrets: The Doctors of the Lower Yangzi Region and Popular Gynecology in Late Imperial China" (Yale University) that forms the basis of her forthcoming book.

pathological problems. In the 2002 article, her study of ghost fetuses and problematic pregnancies reveals the intriguing question of diagnostic uncertainty about pregnancy in Ming-Qing texts, as well as new etiological analyses of such phenomena by Ming-Qing doctors. Such uncertainty made space for negotiation between female patients, with their subjective narrative of their own bodily experience based on language specific to the Ming-Qing social and cultural context, and male doctors, with their long, rich tradition of *fuke* learning in its own technical idiom. Clearly, like Furth and Duden, Wu attempts to show the significance of medicine and the female body in late imperial China as a case of an alternative understanding of the body before modern biomedicine dominated our sensitivity, numbed our imagination, and monopolized our language about the body.

Besides the contributions of Lee and Wu on early, Sui-Tang, and late imperial medicine and women, there are also works that are not entirely on medicine but are closely related to the question of the cultural meaning of the female body, especially in regard to bodily techniques. Here the works of Francesca Bray, Dorothy Ko, and again Li Jianmin should be mentioned. In her book on gender and technology, Bray describes abortion and menstrual regulation as gynotechnics, or embodied practices that upper-class Chinese women skillfully manipulated to control their reproductive activities in order to achieve ideal womanhood or enhance their social role of the *mater*.[19] While Bray relies essentially on printed medical cases of the late imperial period as sources, reflecting the importance of printing in the circulation of medical knowledge for elite women, other authors, such as Liu Jingzhen 劉靜貞and Li Bozhong 李伯重, emphasize the popular, often oral tradition in the diffusion of the techniques of abortion and contraception in post-Song China. Even though their concerns are more social or even demographic, their studies fully reveal that the wide spread of medical knowledge and bodily techniques among women since the Song, often independent of the development of the print culture, allowed them to have much greater control of their own reproductive bodies than one could have imagined, often to the disadvantage of the patriarchal line.[20] Ko's

[19] Francesca Bray, *Technology and Gender: Fabrics of Power in Late Imperial China* (Berkeley: University of California Press, 1995), 334.

[20] Liu Jingzhen, "Cong shun zi huai tai di baoying chuanshuo kan Song dai funü di shengyu wenti" 從損子壞胎的報應傳說看宋代婦女的生育問題, *Dalu zazhi* 大陸雜誌 90.1 (1995):24-39; Li Bozhong, "Duotai, biyun yu jueyu—Song-Yuan-

study of footbinding in imperial China focuses on the body "as attire," an idea obviously inspired by the notion of the body as having fluid and negotiable boundaries as demonstrated by Duden and Furth.[21] Ko's point becomes all the more intriguing when Furth observes in a Ming medical text that the bound foot was identified as "a genital zone of the body."[22] One other interesting bodily technique that has somewhat escaped the attention of scholars of the later imperial period was the women's use of charm to attract men. Li Jianmin described the use of drugs and magic by women in early China in the "art of charming men" (*meidao* 媚道) to gain or retain the love of men. Techniques for "charming" men and for producing a male heir were two main aspects of the early art of the bedchamber for women.[23] It is hard to imagine that such techniques would fall out of fashion in the later imperial period; rather, such knowledge, like that on birth control and footbinding, was not systematically recorded in printed medical texts and should be looked for in other kinds of documents.

On the other hand, the development of another intriguing technique of the female body in the late imperial period, inner alchemy (*nü jindan* 女金丹), was apparently more closely related to the publishing industry. While Furth discusses this technique as a problematic and esoteric religious practice contradictory to the ideal Confucian female body as a robust performer of reproductive functions, Elena Valussi, in a recent doctoral dissertation drawing on printed handbooks about the technique, suggests that this Daoist practice was in fact a "complex and multifaceted phenomenon."[24] According to Valussi, the potentially subversive consequences of the practice (stopping of the menses, resulting in a nonreproductive female body) could be counterbalanced by conservative social behavioral norms imposed on

---

Ming-Qing shiji Jiang-Zhe diqu di jieyu fangfa ji qi yunyong yu chuanbuo" 墮胎、避孕與絕育—宋元明清時期江浙地區的節育方法及其運用與傳播 *Zhongguo xueshu* 中國學術 1 (2000):71-99.

[21] Dorothy Ko, "The Body as Attire: The Shifting Meanings of Footbinding in 17th-Century China," *Journal of Women's History*, 8 (1997):8-27; and her more recent work, *Every Step a Lotus: Shoes for Bound Feet* (Berkeley: University of California Press, 2001).

[22] Furth, *A Flourishing Yin*, 168.

[23] Li Jianmin, "Furen meidao kao: chuantong jiating di chongtu yu huajie fangshu"「婦人媚道」考— 傳統家庭的衝突與化解方術, *Xinshixue* 7.4 (1996):1-32.

[24] Elena Valussi, "Beheading the Red Dragon: A History of Female Inner Alchemy in Late Imperial China" (Ph.D. diss., SOAS University of London, 2003). See the "Conclusion" of this thesis.

female practitioners by male collators of the handbooks. Moreover, the subversiveness of the technique varied according to the age, social and religious status, and even occupation of the practicing women. The technique could even be seen as a "practice that centered on the stabilization and refinement of menstruation" along the line of Bray's argument.[25] In other words, social, religious, and medical norms interplayed in extremely complex ways on the female body in the late imperial and modern periods, further complicating the conceptualization of the gendered body and thus calling for further research in this area.

While studies on bodily techniques practiced essentially by women, including abortion, infanticide, and other techniques that deterred reproduction, seem to support the challenging argument of James Lee and Wang Feng that Chinese reproductive culture produced fertility restraint within marriage, thus having a long-term effect on demographic change,[26] other aspects of medicine for women in the late imperial period are likely to suggest very different conclusions. The persistent concern about the well-being of the reproductive body, male and female alike—as shown in medical texts of Confucian doctors of the late imperial period, such as Wang Ji, discussed by Grant and Hanson in this issue; the changing ideas of "nourishing life" that condemned the restraint of ejaculation; and the reinforcement of the procreative duty imposed on the head of household that "took unquestioned priority over the body's other uses and aspirations," as described by Furth[27]—remind us that ensuring the proliferation of offspring remained a major preoccupation of doctors and their patients. It is difficult at this point to make broad generalizations about the significance of various bodily techniques on demographic changes in the late imperial period. Other factors must be taken into account, such as differences between periods and regions, ethnic or religious groups, and socioeconomic situations.

Another relevant topic that has been studied recently is the role of female practitioners of medicine, including healers, midwives, drug sellers, and so on. Both Furth and Lee have treated the topic in their respective historical periods, and I addressed this subject in

[25] Furth, *A Flourishing Yin*, 219-20. Valussi, "Beheading the Red Dragon," Ch. 5.

[26] James Z. Lee and Wang Feng, *One Quarter of Humanity: Malthusian Mythology and Chinese Realities* (Cambridge, Mass.: Harvard University Press, 1999), esp. 90-99.

[27] Furth, *A Flourishing Yin*, 202-4.

regard to the late imperial period in an article published in 1999 in the book announcing the launching of this journal.[28] That article stresses the discrepancy between the dominant discourse on the evil influence of unskilled and immoral female healers and the importance of their real social role, especially in a culture of strict gender segregation. While the anxiety provoked by unruly women penetrating the boundaries between the inner and outer social space was increasing in the late imperial period, there was at the same time an interesting development of respectable female literati well versed in medicine, of whom Tan Yunxian 談允賢 (sixteenth century) was a most remarkable figure. Furth has a long section discussing her work and healing principles, and another important Chinese historian of medicine, Zheng Jinsheng 鄭金生 published an article on Tan and her achievements, also in 1999.[29] This article provides a useful summary of Tan's medical work, especially her skill in acupuncture and moxa, and points out her accomplishments as a document of social history of the late Ming.

While interests in cultural and social studies of medicine and gender continue to grow, especially in America and Taiwan, research on the history of *fuke* with a more traditional and positivist approach continues in China. After Ma Dazheng's book was published in 1991, Zhang Zhibin, a younger scholar, published her first book on the history of *fuke* disorders in 2000,[30] based on her doctoral dissertation defended in Beijing in 1998. Like Ma's work, Zhang's book traces the development of *fuke* pathology from pre-imperial to late imperial times. It is interesting to note the strong conviction she takes in "revealing the true face of history" in writing this book, a position that inevitably makes the result very different from present-day Western research and even that done in Taiwan. As revealed in the review by Mak in this issue, the author clearly takes a clinical approach to the question by discussing what she defines as gynecological disorders and their medical or technical treatment in each historical period.

---

[28] Angela Ki Che Leung, "Women Practicing Medicine in Premodern China," in H. Zurndorfer, ed. *Chinese Women in the Imperial Past: New Perspectives* (Leiden: Brill, 1999), 101-34.
On this topic, one should also mention an older article by Victoria Cass, "Female Healers in the Ming and the Lodge of Ritual and Ceremony," *Journal of the American Oriental Society* 106 (1986): 233-40.

[29] Zheng Jinsheng, "Mingdai nüyi Tan Yunxian ji qi yi'an 'Nüyi zayan'" 明代女醫談允賢及其醫案『女醫雜言』*Zhonghua yishi zazhi* 中華醫史雜誌 29.3 (1999):153-56.

[30] See note 4.

She is sensitive to the appearance of "new" names and categories of disorders, which she often uses as an important measure to evaluate the development of the discipline.

The most interesting difference between this book and those by some of her predecessors is that she places less importance on the development of Song *fuke,* which she groups together with that in the Jin and Yuan periods. Even though she admits the originality of the focus on "Blood as the leader" in Song medical gynecology, she considers it a heritage from the Tang medical learning, especially that of Sun Simiao. Moreover, she seems to have a much higher opinion of *fuke* in the Ming-Qing than in the Song, her reasons being "the classification of the diseases becomes equitable [*sic*], the naming becomes appropriate, the ideas are clear and more content is added. On causes, [the] doctors paid attention to the internal ones...and criticized some views [that] diseases may be brought by ghosts and gods."[31] I do not intend to criticize this book for its positivist approach, but simply to show the numerous layers of meanings that one can retrieve in old medical texts on woman's body and the many research possibilities that one can still locate in this field. In fact, many of Zhang's findings do not differ from those of the authors mentioned above, yet her very different interpretations and conclusions provide an interesting perspective for further musing and reflection.

One last point that should be raised here is that there is relatively little interest among Japanese scholars in the history of Chinese medicine for women. Related to this point, the latest publication of Lee Jen-der is revealing.[32] In this article on the earliest extant Japanese medical work, *Ishinpo* 醫心方 (Recipes of the heart of medicine), dating to 982, Lee shows how the Japanese compiler Tana Yasuyori 丹波康賴 (912-95) selected from early Chinese medical classics only those discussions related to childbirth in sections on medicine for women, and leaving out those on other bodily disorders. The compiler was obviously more interested in the strictly gestational aspect of the female body—not surprising as the book's readers were essentially male aristocrats concerned with the reproduction of heirs. What

[31] Zhang, *Gudai zhongyi fuchanke jibing shi* (English summary, 424).

[32] Lee, "'*Ishinpo'* lun 'furen zhubing suoyou' ji qi xiangguan wenti." Readers of this *Nan Nü* issue may note that there are other acceptable spellings for Tana and his publication: Tanba, Tanba no Yasuyori, or Tamba; or *Ishinpō*, *Ishimpō*. We will use here Tana Yasuyori, *Ishinpo* throughout this issue.

is more intriguing is that after the publication of *Ishinpo,* the first full Japanese gynecological work was not published until the mid-sixteenth century, with a few obstetrical works printed during the fourtheenth and fifteenth centuries.[33] That was three centuries after the publication of Chen Ziming's classic in China. Lee concludes that traditional Japanese doctors did not study the female body with the same meticulous obsession as did Chinese doctors. This point may also be reflected in the relative lack of interest among Japanese academics for traditional Chinese medicine for women. Many important contributions have been made by serious Japanese historians of Chinese medicine in the philosophy of medicine, the nature of *qi*, the art of "nourishing life," alchemy, pharmacopeia (*bencao* 本草), Daoism and medicine, and so on, but, until now, almost no notable research on *fuke* and medicine for women even in broad terms has been published, not even as part of a more general history of medicine.[34]

Conclusion

Recent publications on medicine for women in China show that this topic defines a field of scholarly research of great potential. Discussions are not limited to strictly medical questions, but are inevitably related to specific social contexts and to the cultural and intellectual developments of imperial China. Both traditional or sinological and cultural approaches are possible for analysis of relevant questions, and often researchers tend to rely on both to produce more exciting results. So far, we have only talked about research done on imperial China, and there are, in my opinion, even greater possibilities on the modern period when China faced challenges from Western medicine and culture. While the confrontation between Chinese and Western medicine has been studied by a number of talented young scholars,[35] there have been few serious studies related specifically to

[33] Lee, "'*Ishinpo*' lun 'furen zhubing suoyou' ji qi xiangguan wenti," 503-5.

[34] Important Japanese scholars of the history of science and medicine such as Ishida Hidemi 石田秀實, Sakade Yoshinobu 板出祥伸, Yamada Keiji 山田慶兒, Morita Denichiro 森田傳一郎, et al., have written important works on various aspects of Chinese medicine, but none so far has shown any particular interest in the history of *fuke per se*. Their rare and typically brief mentioning of *fuke* is often only a minor illustration of the main topics of medicine that they study in depth.

[35] Such as Sean Hsiang-lin Lei 雷祥麟,"When Chinese Medicine Encountered the State 1910-1949" (Ph.D. diss., University of Chicago, 1999); and his "How Did

the development of modern Chinese gynecology.[36] The changes in or the "Westernization" of the conceptualization of the female body in China, in medical, sociopolitical, and cultural terms should be a most fruitful topic of research, and hopefully we shall not wait for too long to see work done on this period.

Chinese Medicine Become Experiential? The Political Epistemology of *Jingyan,*" *Positions* 10.2 (2002):334-64; and Bridie Andrews, "The Making of Modern Chinese Medicine, 1895-1937" (Ph.D. diss., Cambridge University, 1996), and her "Tuberculosis and the Assimilation of Germ Theory in China, 1895-1937," *Journal of the History of Medicine and Allied Sciences* 52 (1997):114-57.

[36] I can think of only two, Frank Dikotter's *Imperfect Conceptions: Medical Knowledge, Birth Defects, and Eugenics in China* (New York: Columbia University Press, 1998), and his *Sex, Culture, and Modernity in China: Medical Science and the Construction of Sexual Identities in the Early Republican Period* (Honolulu: University of Hawaii Press, 1995).

MEDICINE FOR WOMEN IN EARLY CHINA: A PRELIMINARY SURVEY

BY

ROBIN D. S. YATES
(McGill University)

Abstract

This study reviews aspects of the history of medicine for women from approximately the third century BCE to the tenth century CE. It focuses on therapies during the months of pregnancy and childbirth as recorded in newly discovered texts, on the developing pharmacopeia, and on ritual procedures. It argues that acupuncture was used only rarely on pregnant women and that many cultural and religious beliefs and practices, including those drawn from the Buddhist, Daoist, and popular traditions, influenced procedures undertaken in preparation for and during the birth process.

Introduction[1]

In this essay, I wish to consider some of the many issues relating to the development of medicine for women in the period prior to 960, noting at the outset that in traditional Chinese medicine, *fu* 婦 in the

[1] This paper was first presented to the Department of East Asian Languages and Literatures and the Women's Studies Program, Yale University. I would like to express my deep gratitude to Professors Kang-i Sun Chang and Margaret Homans for extending their generous invitation. It was subsequently presented at the University of Durham: I would like to thank Dr. Daria Berg for the opportunity to discuss the issues with her and her colleagues and students. I would also like to thank the three anonymous reviewers for their exceptionally careful reading of the first two drafts of the essay. They provided me with most valuable comments, guided me on a number of crucial issues, and helped me avoid several mistakes. Needless to say, I am solely responsible for the opinions expressed in this final version and for the errors that remain. Vivienne Lo and Christopher Cullen generously sent me a copy of their excellent new book *Medieval Chinese Medicine: The Dunhuang Medical Manuscripts* (London: Routledge Curzon, 2005), which is directly relevant to the latter portion of this article. Unfortunately, however, I received it too late to incorporate the findings of the various chapters into the body of this essay. I shall only refer the reader to certain chapters in my footnotes.

term *fuke* 婦科 (gynecology) always referred to a married woman: girls were not considered to be gendered and were included in the category of children (*yinger* 嬰兒).[2] Therefore in this article I am not going to review the history of the medicine used to treat the ailments of prepubescent girls or unmarried adult women, such as nuns,[3] nor am I going to discuss women as healers in their own right.[4] This

---

[2] As far as I am aware, among Western scholars, only Charlotte Furth, "From Birth to Birth: The Growing Body in Chinese Medicine," in Anne Behnke Kinney, ed., *Chinese Views of Childhood* (Honolulu: University of Hawaii Press, 1995), 172-83, has explored the rich sources available for the study of the history of Chinese pediatrics. In Chinese, Li Zhende 李貞德 (Lee Jen-der), has revealed many important facets of women's medicine in the first millennium CE. See her articles "Han Tang zhijian yishu zhong de shengchan zhi dao" 漢唐之間醫書中的生產之道, *Bulletin of the Institute of History and Philology* 中央研究院歷史語言研究所集刊 67.3 (1996): 533-654, and "Han Tang zhijian qiuzi yifang shitan—jianlun fuke lanshang yu xingbie lunshu" 漢唐之間求子醫方試探—兼論婦科濫觴與性別論述 *Bulletin of the Institute of History and Philology* 68.2 (1997):283-367.

[3] Tana Yasuyori 丹波康賴, *Ishinpo* 醫心方; I have used the edition published in Zhao Mingshan 趙明山 et al., eds., (Shenyang: Liaoning kexue jishu chubanshe, 1996), 3, 21.862, section 29, "Zhi furen yunan fang" 治婦人欲男方 (Prescriptions for a woman who desires a man), may be providing treatment for such a man-less, frustrated, woman in the following passage:

> The *Daqing jing* states: "The August Emperor asked a question of the Plain Woman (Su Nü 素女) and she replied: 'When a woman is 28 or 29 or 23 or 24, her *yinqi* is abundant, and she desires to have a man and she cannot control herself. She eats and drinks without tasting [what she consumes. i.e., there is no taste to what she eats or drinks], all her pulses move in her body, she feels a repletion in her essence and her pulses, fluid leaks out and soils her clothes, in her vagina there are insects like horsetails, three *fen* 分 [three-tenths of an inch *cun* 寸] long; those with red heads are irritating, and those with black heads produce froth.
>
> "The prescription for curing her is: Make a penis out of dough as long or short, large or small as is appropriate, dip it in pure rice spirits [*jiangqing*] twice. Wrap it with silk floss and insert it into the vagina and touch the insects as it goes in and out. Take it out and then insert it again just as though she was having a man. When there are many insects, there are thirty [of them]; when there are few, there are twenty."
> 大清經云皇帝問素女對曰女人年廿八九若廿三四陰氣盛欲得男子不能自禁食飲無味,百脉動體,候精脉實,汁出污衣裳,女人陰中有蟲如馬尾,長三分,赤頭者悶,黑頭者沫治之方用麵作玉莖,長短大小隨意,以醬清及二辨綿裹之納陰中蟲即着來出出復納如得大夫其蟲多者卅少者廿

I have not had access to the Japanese original of Tamba's work. See also Michel Strickmann (Bernard Faure, ed.), *Chinese Magical Medicine* (Stanford: Stanford University Press, 2002), 245.

[4] For a brief discussion of the few references to female doctors in the Han specializing in women's medicine, see Ma Dazheng 馬大正, *Zhongguo fuchanke fazhan shi* 中國婦產科發展史 (Xian: Shaanxi kexue jiaoyu chubanshe, 1991), 37; for women as midwives and healers from the Song to the Qing, see Angela Ki Che Leung, "Women Practicing Medicine in Premodern China," in Harriet Zurndorfer, ed., *Chinese Women in the Imperial Past: New Perspectives* (Leiden: Brill, 1999), 101-34; for

would lead us to a consideration of women as shamans, midwives, and wet nurses, all fascinating topics, but beyond the scope of the present endeavor.[5] I shall review some of the texts recently discovered by archaeologists dating from the Qin and Han dynasties that relate to medicine for women and will consider especially the interface between medicine and ritual in birthing practices, paying attention to the management of polluting substances produced by the mother. I will argue that medicine for women in the pre-Song period was influenced by a wide range of cultural and religious beliefs and practices and that these must be taken into consideration when assessing medicine for women as it developed into the complex discipline of gynecology that it became from Song times on.

First of all, to put this study in context, Charlotte Furth argues that a fully theorized medicine for women "developed into a mature system of gynecology in the Song dynasty" (960-1268).[6] Literate, usually male, doctors identified themselves as experts in gynecology and wrote texts specifically devoted to the subject. A typical, and influential, figure was Chen Ziming 陳自明 (ca. 1190-1270) of the Southern Song, whose *Furen liangfang* 婦人良方 (Excellent prescriptions for women) (1237) is a rich repository of contemporary knowledge about medicine for women.[7] Second, gynecology was

women as lay healers in late imperial fiction, see Daria Berg, *Perceptions of Lay Healers in Late Imperial China*, Durham East Asian Papers 15 (Durham: Department of East Asian Studies, University of Durham, 2000); and for "grannies" in the Ming, see Victoria Cass, *Dangerous Women: Warriors, Grannies and Geisha of the Ming* (Lanham, Md.: Rowman and Littlefield, 1999), Ch. 3, 47-64. Sima Qian 司馬遷, *Shiji* 史記, "Biography of Bian Que" 扁鵲列傳 (Beijing: Zhonghua shuju, 1985), *ce* 9, 105.2794, states that when Bian Que visited the city of Handan 邯鄲 where women were valued, he became a gynecologist, literally "a doctor [of illnesses] below the belt" (*daixia yi* 帶下醫). While the historical reality of Bian Que is in much dispute, Sima's notice suggests that there were specialists in women's illnesses associated with pregnancy as early as the Warring States Period. Duan Chengshi 段成式 (died 863) reports that acupuncture and herbal doctors made offerings at Bian's tomb east of Lucheng 盧城 in the Wei dynasty (220-65), and therefore they were called "Lu doctors" 盧醫, but Duan does not indicate whether these included doctors who were specialists in women's medicine. See *Youyang zazu* 酉陽雜俎, "Qian ji" 前集 (Beijing: Zhonghua shuju, 1981), 7.73.

[5] See, *inter alia*, Lee Jen-der's article "Wet Nurses in Early Imperial China," *Nan Nü: Men, Women and Gender in Early and Imperial China* 2.1 (2000): 1-39.

[6] Charlotte Furth, *A Flourishing Yin: Gender in China's Medical History, 960-1665* (Berkeley: University of California Press, 1999), 60.

[7] Chen Ziming, *Furen liangfang jiaozhu buyi* 婦人良方校注補遺, supplement by Xiong Zongli 熊宗立 of the Ming and commentary by Xue Ji 薛己 of the Ming (Shanghai: Shanghai kexue jishu chubanshe, 1991).

institutionalized at the imperial court and in the Imperial Medical Bureau, where state medical training was organized into nine separate departments, of which gynecology and pediatrics were two.[8] It would appear that gynecology, like other medical specialties, was the subject of examinations for testing the qualifications of those wishing to practice as official medical experts.[9] Third, and most important, was the systematization of the discipline whereby, in Furth's words, there was an "application to women's disorders of a paradigm of diagnosis that made it easier to relate diverse symptoms to holistic body functions."[10]

Song gynecology, Furth argues, participated in the general emphasis on innovation in medical discourses that sought to provide integrated and consistent explanations for diseases. Specifically, she demonstrates that, over three centuries, Song doctors, building on the numerous therapies and suggestions transmitted to them from earlier times, especially the notion that in women "Blood was the leader" taken from the work of the Sui and early Tang doctor Sun Simo 孫思邈 (581-682?), and using what she calls "pattern diagnosis" (*bianzheng* 辨證),[11] reduced the vast number of symptoms observed by themselves and their predecessors "into a smaller number of broad categories that could in turn be related to each other dynamically."[12] Standardized into eight rubrics, symptoms were seen to possess a '"root" (*ben* 本) pattern identified with some combination of yin/yang, cold/hot, inner/outer or depletion/repletion factors," and doctors then organized their wide array of prescriptions so that they were linked to underlying internal disorders "now seen as gendered forms of illness."[13] Doctors became particularly interested in

---

[8] Furth, *A Flourishing Yin*, 66.

[9] The Song government was generally activist in its orientation and established, among other institutions, pharmacies throughout the country, one of whose functions was to dispense prescriptions to the population in times of epidemic.

[10] Furth, *A Flourishing Yin*, 63.

[11] In a personal communication, Charlotte Furth wishes to emphasize what she wrote in *A Flourishing Yin*, 65, n. 16, that *bianzheng* is a modern term. The Song term was *bian* 辨, the *locus classicus* being in the work of Kou Zongshi 寇宗奭 (eleventh-twelfth centuries), *Bencao yanyi* 本草衍義 (Elucidation of the meaning of pharmaceutics) (*Xuxiu siku quanshu* 續修四庫全書 [Shanghai: Shanghai guji chubanshe, 1995-99], 990). For the translation of this passage, see Paul U. Unschuld, *Medicine in China: A History of Pharmaceutics* (Berkeley: University of California Press, 1986), 93-94.

[12] Furth, *A Flourishing Yin*, 65.

[13] Furth, *A Flourishing Yin*, 66.

regulating menstruation and developed concern about parturition.

Prior to the Song, from the Han dynasty on (late third century BCE to the beginning of the third century CE), Furth argues, the body was conceived of in medical discourses as being "genuinely androgynous,"[14] and she coins the term "the Yellow Emperor's body" to describe its *yin-yang* characteristics.[15] She states that "[i]n the early imperial era [the] clinical tradition [of *fuke*, gynecology], invisible in the account of the Yellow Emperor's body, . . . was an eclectic one, incorporating herbal drinks, medicinal pastes and washes, poultices and heat treatments, massage, moxibustion and acupuncture, ritual and diet, transmitted in manuscript traditions independent of midwifery."[16] Her argument revealing how the Chinese body came to be fully gendered in the Song, as was Chinese traditional medicine as a whole, needless to say, has enormous implications for our understanding of the development of the patriarchal social and ideological system of imperial China.[17]

Concerned with analyzing the changes that took place in the Song and later times, Furth does not clarify for the reader the relationships that the various early, pre-Song, therapies had to each other and whether there were any changes in medical practices over time. In this paper, I shall examine medicine for women in the pre-Song period, for I cannot do justice to the complexity of Furth's arguments for the Song and later dynasties. However, I believe that the fact that medicine was institutionalized in the Song is much less significant for her thesis than her analysis of Song doctors' understanding of the etiology of diseases, for the state's attempt at controlling the training and distribution of drugs and the assignment of physicians, whether specialists in gynecology or in other fields, was

---

[14] Furth, *A Flourishing Yin*, 52.

[15] See also Lisa Raphals, *Sharing the Light: Representations of Women and Virtue in Early China* (Albany: State University of New York Press, 1998), Ch. 7, "Yin-Yang in Medical Texts"; and Manfred Porkert, *Theoretical Foundations of Chinese Medicine: Systems of Correspondence* (Cambridge, Mass.: MIT Press, 1978), 9-43.

[16] Furth, *A Flourishing Yin*, 60.

[17] Furth notes in *A Flourishing Yin* that "Chinese medical thought never abandoned the vision of bodily androgyny, but with twists and turns returned to it again and again" (306). With great insight, she raises the question why in medical theory "bodily gender was a plastic androgyny, while social gender was based on fixed hierarchy?" (305). This fascinating contradiction deserves to be studied in an extensive research program; I shall not attempt to answer it in this preliminary review of early medicine for women.

abandoned in later dynasties after the Song collapsed in the face of the Mongol invasion.

The "Yellow Emperor's Body" and the Medicine of Systematic Correspondence

Furth's chapter on the "Yellow Emperor's body" provides a dense, abstract, theoretically sophisticated and complex discussion of how the qualities and relational logic of the multivalent and complementary concepts of *yin* and *yang*, as manifested in the natural world and in human bodies through the medium of *qi* 氣, were manipulated by Chinese doctors both in their theoretical discussions of difference and in their functional applications of the concepts in therapy and, metaphorically and symbolically, in the way that they related male and female bodies to the cosmos as a whole.

Nevertheless, we may say from the point of view of a more concrete understanding of difference, that both the male and the female body had *yin* and *yang* aspects. In this characterization, what was hidden, such as the internal organs, was *yin*, whereas what was outer, such as the skin, was *yang*. The front was *yang* and the back was *yin*. The left side was *yang* and the right side *yin*. The top half of the body was *yang*, the lower parts, especially the genitals, were *yin*. As Furth points out, "the generative functions" were associated with Kidney and Water, the most *yin* of the Five Phases, and also the "generative vitalities" were "rooted . . . in a Vital Gate (*ming men* 命門) and Cinnabar Field (*dan tian* 丹田) located somewhere beneath the navel in all human beings. The Vital Gate also had an indistinct morphological association with Kidney. Here concentrated primordial aspects of reproductive vitality deeper than visible male or female genitals or functions, and associated with primordial *qi* itself."[18] Chinese doctors were not interested in anatomy, in contrast to Western doctors from Renaissance times on. Hua Tuo 華佗 (second to third centuries) was the only physician in the later Han or Jin dynasties said to have actually examined internal organs and treated an abdominal mass by excision.[19] However, he was unique,

[18] Furth, *A Flourishing Yin*, 29.

[19] The *Lingshu jing* 靈樞經 (Canon of the divine pivot) has a section, 31, on the intestines and stomach in which the size of the teeth and tongue and dimensions and capacity of both intestines and stomach are given. This suggests that doctors had measured these organs with some precision. See Ren Jiyu 任繼愈, ed., *Zhongguo*

and although he is promoted now as great scientist, much of what is attributed to him may not be historically accurate.[20]

So the early Chinese body was conceived of as consisting of skin, bones, and flesh (not muscles),[21] through which circulation tracts of *qi* and Blood traversed, linking extremities (head, fingers, toes, limbs) with internal organs. Internal organs or viscera were only vaguely described. These were seen to be ensembles of functions, not structures, and imagined as officials in charge of their respective systems. As a consequence, in the grand Han synthesis created by male literati doctors, what Paul Unschuld calls the "medicine of systematic correspondence,"[22] they were correlated with similarly named of-

---

kexue jishu dianji tonghui 中國科學技術典籍通彙 (Zhengzhou: Henan jiaoyu chubanshe, 1994), "Yixue," 醫學 *juan* 1, 377-78. The knowledge is used to determine how long it would take for a person to die if he did not eat grain (section 32, 378). Qin legal texts discovered at Shuihudi, Hubei, in 1975 show that autopsies were performed in the Qin in the third century BCE. See Katrina C. D. McLeod and Robin D. S. Yates, "Forms of Ch'in Law: An Annotated Translation of the *Feng-chen shih*," *Harvard Journal of Asiatic Studies* 41.1 (1981):111-63. But this legal practice does not seem to have led to an interest in examining, weighing, and evaluating the internal organs *per se*. In this collection, there is one case of a bondservant (*liqie* 隸妾) who had given birth a number of times being ordered by the Qin government authorities to inspect a woman who had a miscarriage as a result of fight with another woman. The bondservant washed in a bowl of water a mass of blood as big as a hand that had been expelled and concluded that indeed it was a fetus, with head, body, arms, fingers, legs, and toes, even though the eyes, ears, and nose, and sex could not be determined.

[20] For his biographies, see *Hou Hanshu* 後漢書 (Beijing: Zhonghua shuju, 1982) *ce* 10, 82B.2736-41, and *Sanguozhi* 三國志 (*Weishu* 魏書) (Beijing: Zhonghua shuju, 1973), *ce* 3, 29.799-806, in which he is recorded as correctly diagnosing two cases in which a fetus had died in the womb and was causing serious discomfit and illness. See Li Jingwei 李經緯 and Lin Zhaogeng 林昭庚, eds., *Zhongguo yixue tongshi* 中國醫學通史, "Gudai juan" 古代卷 (Beijing: Renmin weisheng chubanshe, 2000), 137. It is clear that surgery was but one of the techniques Hua used, and many texts in various disciplines were later attributed to him. See also Zhao Pushan 趙璞珊, *Zhongguo gudai yixue* 中國古代醫學 (Beijing: Zhonghua shuju, 1997), 55-57; and Li Jingwei, "Surgery in Ancient China," in Institute of the History of Natural Sciences, Chinese Academy of Sciences, ed., *Ancient China's Technology and Science* (Beijing: Foreign Languages Press, 1983), 369-71.

[21] See Shigehisa Kuriyama's recent book *The Expressiveness of the Body and the Divergence of Greek and Chinese Medicine* (New York: Zone Books, 1999), Ch. 3, "Muscularity and Identity," 111-51, for the emergence of the notion of "muscles" and their visual representation in the West. Muscles were, however, certainly recognized in military medicine, a subject that I am treating elsewhere (*Science and Civilisation in China*, vol. 5, Part 8, in preparation). See Robin D. S. Yates, "History of Chinese Military Medicine" (Paper Presented at the Conference of the Society of Military History, University of Calgary, May 24-27, 2001).

[22] Paul U. Unschuld, *Medicine in China: A History of Ideas* (Berkeley: University of California Press, 1985).

ficials in the macrocosm both in the civil bureaucracy, and in the cosmos as a whole, in the heavens. Heaven, Earth, and Man were understood as homologies of each other and dependent on each other. As the *Huangdi neijing suwen* 黃帝內經素問 (Plain questions from the Yellow Emperor's canon of internal medicine) puts it:

> The Yellow Emperor said, "Now from ancient times [*qi*] is what penetrates heaven, is the root of life, and is rooted in *yin* and *yang*. Between Heaven and Earth, in the six directions, everything from the nine provinces and the nine bodily orifices to the five visceral systems and the twelve joints, is penetrated by the *qi* of heaven. Alive [it manifests itself in] the Five [Phases] and its *qi* are three. If these numbers are opposed, then heteropathic *qi* harms people. This is the root of long life."[23]
> 黃帝曰:夫自古通天者,生之本,本於陰陽,天地之間,六合之內,其氣九州九竅五臟十二節,皆通乎天氣.其生五,其氣三,數犯此者則邪氣傷人,此壽命之本也.

Thus in acupuncture theory developed in the Han, the cosmic *qi* was also believed to enter and exit the body through certain "holes" or "caverns" (*xue* 穴) along the circulation tracts, hence the therapy of applying needles to influence the flow or stagnation of the internal *qi* in those tracts.[24] The body had to be kept open through the skin and the nine bodily orifices to allow for the movement of *qi* in and out, by which sustenance was maintained. Wastes were to be expelled, and heteropathic (bad) *qi* flowing through the external world was to be kept out and good *qi* ingested and circulated through the body, consciously and unconsciously. Blockages in the movement of internal *qi* as well as the attack and entry of external heteropathic *qi* were thought to bring on disease. This was true for both men and women.

It has been argued that the medicine of systematic correspondence gradually superseded, especially among the male intellectual elite,

---

[23] "Sheng qi tongtian lun" 生氣通天論 (Treatise on how live *qi* penetrates heaven). See Shandong Zhongyi xueyuan 山東醫學院 and Hebei Yixueyuan 河北醫學院, eds., *Huangdi neijing suwen jiaoshi* 黃帝內經素問校釋 (Beijing: Renmin weisheng chubanshe, 1995), *pian 3*, 1.28-29. There are different interpretations of the "three *qi*." Either they are the *qi* of Heaven, of Earth, and of Man, the opinion of Wang Bing 王冰 (fl. 762), or they are the *qi* of *yin* and *yang* that each divide into three, Taiyin 太陰, Shaoyin 少陰 and Queyin 厥陰, and Taiyang 太陽, Shaoyang 少陽, and Yangming 陽明. See Shandong Zhongyi xueyuan and Hebei Yixueyuan, eds., *Huangdi neijing suwen jiaoshi*, 29 n. 6.

[24] Unschuld, *Medicine in China: A History of Ideas*, 71. The most recent study of the origin and development of the theory of circulation tracts is Li Jianmin 李建民, *Sisheng zhi yu: Zhou Qin Han maixue zhi yuanliu* 死生之域：周秦漢脈學之源流 (Taibei: Zhongyang yuan Shiyu suo, 2000).

an earlier medicine based on the more religious notion that disease was caused by ghosts and suprahuman spirits, sometimes referred to as demoniac medicine[25]—in the Shang dynasty, the pregnancies of royal women and the outcome of their labor were the subject of divination[26]—but this latter form of medicine was still pervasive and long lasting in later times, and possessed a wide array of therapies, as Michel Strickmann has documented.[27] Of those therapies in competition with the medicine of systematic correspondence, was there some order to medicine for women in the pre-Song period, or was it just an eclectic assortment of procedures, as Furth seems to suggest it was, and how was medicine for women in early imperial China conceived, and what did it encompass?

Medicine for Women in Recently Discovered Texts

In the bibliography of the Han imperial library created by the Confucian scholars Liu Xiang 劉向(ca. 79-ca. 6 BCE) and his son Liu Xin 劉歆(d. 23), preserved in the *Hanshu* 漢書 compiled in the first century CE by Ban Gu 班固 (32-92) and his famous sister Ban Zhao 班昭 (ca. 49- ca. 120), there is no category of gynecology. This is so even though Liu Xiang was the author of the extremely influential first work of biography of notable women, the *Lienü zhuan* 列女傳, a volume that generated an important tradition of writing about women.[28]

Yet women are not invisible in the Han imperial bibliography. The two Liu's record a book called *Furen yinger fang* 婦人嬰兒方 (Prescriptions for women and infants) in nineteen *juan* (chapters) in the category "Canonical prescriptions or recipes" (*jingfang* 經方), that consists of eleven works with a total of 274 chapters.[29] One of the other

---

[25] For a study of the sources of traditional Chinese medicine, including those available in early times, before the establishment of the paradigm of the medicine of systematic correspondence, see Zhang Canjia 張燦玾, *Zhongyi guji wenxian xue* 中醫古籍文獻學 (Beijing: Renmin weisheng chubanshe, 1998).

[26] Ma Dazheng, *Zhongguo fuchanke fazhan shi*, 5-6.

[27] Strickmann, *Chinese Magical Medicine.*

[28] A number of scholars have been able to trace the changing social position of women and their accompanying values over millennia by analyzing the changing composition of characters, representations, and illustrations in the successive editions of this work. See, for example, Raphals, *Sharing the Light.*

[29] *Hanshu* (Beijing: Zhonghua shuju, 1975), "Yiwen zhi" 藝文志, 30.1777. Women

works listed in the prescriptions section is the *Shen Nong Huangdi shijin* 神農黃帝食禁 (The Divine Husbandman's and the Yellow Emperor's food prohibitions), of the early Han dynasty. As I will discuss later on, food proscriptions played an important part of preparation for giving birth, so it is possible that food taboos and recommendations for women's diet were included in this work, too. Nevertheless, neither of these two works has survived, and it is impossible to determine how they categorized women's illnesses and whether the first text was devoted solely to difficulties, diseases, and treatments relating to pregnancy, childbirth, and the menses, together with recipes for infants and children, or whether it encompassed recipes for female patients for a broader range of illnesses.

Recent archaeological discoveries have given a hint of what the contents of such prescriptions might have been.[30] Two slips, 322 and 323, found among a collection of recipes in tomb 30, Zhoujiatai, of Qin date, indicate that women were to take a different amount of medicine from men in one case for a breathing problem, possibly the result of being bitten by a rabid dog, and, in another, for lumps in the belly. In the latter recipe, it is recommended that the tip of a sword or a *youfang* 有方 halberd be heated and then plunged into strong pure wine (or beer) (*jiu* 酒); this a woman should drink twice seven times, whereas a man should imbibe only seven times.[31]

---

are also present in the "arts of the bedchamber" (*fangzhong* 房中) category; see Douglas Wile, *The Chinese Sexual Yoga Classics Including Women's Solo Meditation Texts* (Albany: State University of New York Press, 1992). Such works were usually written for male practitioners and revealed esoteric practices aimed at achieving immortality; they were not intended for parturient women. However, Li Jianmin, "'Furen meidao kao—chuantong jiating de chongtu yu huajie fangshu" 婦人媚道考—傳統家庭的衝突與化解方術, *Xinshi xue* 新史學 7.4 (1996): 1-30, reprinted in *Fangshu yixue lishi* 方術醫學歷史(Taibei: Nantian shuju, 2000), 95-122, argues that it also included the art of creating a variety of drugs that could be and were administered by women either to "charm" or seduce a lover to show preferential treatment to her or to regain his affection. I do not intend to discuss this tradition in the present paper.

30 Gao Dalun 高大倫, "Juyan Han jian zhong suojian jibing he jibing wenshu kaoshu" 居延漢簡中所見疾病和疾病文書考述, in Gansu sheng wenwu kaogu yanjiusuo 甘肅省文物考古研究所 and Xibei shifan daxue lishi xi 西北師範大學歷史系, eds., *Jiandu xue yanjiu* 簡牘學研究 (Lanzhou: Lanzhou renmin chubanshe, 1997), 2.95, states that no slips relating to gynecology have been found among the documents retrieved by archaeologists, probably because most of the inhabitants of the northwest were young men serving as frontier soldiers. However, records of travelers in the slips indicate that some women did accompany their husbands to their postings.

31 Hubei sheng Jingzhou shi Zhou Liangyu qiao yizhi bowu guan 湖北省荊州市周梁玉橋遺址博物館, ed., *Guanju Qin Han mu jiandu* 關沮秦漢墓簡牘 (Beijing: Zhonghua shuju, 2001), 128-29.

One may presume that here a magical operation is taking place: the sharpness and heat of the sword or halberd, usually used for chopping and killing, is transferred to the beverage which then cures the illness. Since weapons were used to exorcise evil spirits, the disease might have been conceived of, although the text does not say so explicitly, as being caused by demons, or could have been thought to have been brought on by other causes.[32]

Among the wooden slips found in an Eastern Han tomb in the Gobi Desert along the Gansu corridor in northwest China was a double-sided board with two identical prescriptions for unguents for women.[33] The ingredients include:

[gua 栝*] lou* 樓 *Trichosanthes triloba* 3 *sheng* 升
danggui 當歸 *Angelica polymorpha* 10 *fen* 分
baizhi 白茝 (芷) *Angelica anomala* 4 *fen*
fuzi 付子 possibly daughter root *Aconitum autumnale* or *A. carmichaeli*[34] 30 sticks (*mei* 枚)
gancao 甘草 licorice *Glycyrrhiza glabra* 7 *fen*
gongdaiji 弓大鄧 (?) unknown 10 *fen*
gaocao 菒草 (*gaoben* 藁本) *Nothosmyrnium japonicum* 2 *shu* 束

Although it is not possible to determine what this unguent was intended to cure, as Paul Unschuld has pointed out, this prescription and others found in the tomb are complex, combining a number of ingredients in various proportions with various excipients, such

---

[32] Later texts also preserve recipes that call for similar remedies. For example, in the Dunhuang manuscript Stein 3930, Ma Jixing, Wang Shumin 王淑民, Tao Guangzheng 陶廣正, and Fan Feilun 樊飛倫, eds., *Dunhuang yiyao wenxian jijiao* 敦煌醫藥文獻輯校 (Nanjing: Jiangsu guji chubanshe, 1998), section 29, Anonymous Medical Prescriptions 10, 390, it is recommended to heat a large axe head until it is red hot, put it in wine, and then drink the concoction to cure pains in the stomach after childbirth. For a brief description of this Dunhuang manuscript, see Wang Shumin, "Abstracts of the Medical Manuscripts from Dunhuang," item 31, Appendix 2, in Vivienne Lo and Christopher Cullen, eds., *Medieval Chinese Medicine*, 407-08.

[33] Gansu sheng bowuguan 甘肅省博物館 and Wuwei xian wenhua guan 武威縣文化館, eds., *Wuwei Handai yijian* 武威漢代醫簡 (Beijing: Wenwu chubanshe, 1975), 17-18, slips 88A and 88B; see also Zhang Shouren 張壽仁, "Yijian biji" 醫簡筆記, *Jiandu xuebao* 簡牘學報 17 (1999): 224-25. For a general discussion of Han dynasty medical records found in the northwest desert, see Xie Guihua 謝桂華, translated by Vivienne Lo, "Han Bamboo and Wooden Medical Records Discovered in Military Sites from the North-western Frontier Regions," in Lo and Cullen, *Medieval Chinese Medicine*, 78-106.

[34] Zhang Xiancheng 張顯成, *Jianbo yaoming yanjiu* 簡帛藥名研究 (Xian: Xian shifan daxue chubanshe, 1997, 106-09.

as lard—as in the case of the unguent for women—, honey, milk, and cheese made from camel's milk.[35] The prescriptions found in the Western Han tomb at Mawangdui 馬王堆 in Changsha, south of the Yangzi River, dating from 168 BCE, that contain no specific recommendations for women also follow this form, but also include magical formulas and instructions on the correct timing of therapy and drug ingestion.[36] The practice of combining drugs with different therapeutic values in different proportions reveals that they were based on centuries of prior experience with the therapeutic properties of drugs from many different sources.[37] In fact, a number of the Wuwei ingredients, including *Trichosanthes*, the two angelicas, the daughter root, and licorice, remained important herbal drugs for use in gynecology, as well as in general therapy, right up to the present day, two thousand years later, so this unguent may have been intended to be massaged into the skin of a pregnant woman to cure some unnamed gynecological disorder.

It is also worth mentioning that at the beginning of May 1999, the tomb of Wu Yang 吳陽, Marquis of Yuanling of the Han, who died in 162 BCE, was discovered in Yuanling County, Hunan. Among the tomb's rich contents is a text called "Recipes for Fine Food" (*Meishi fang* 美食方).[38] This important discovery was reported at a conference held in the summer of 2000, but only very brief excerpts of the texts were revealed, and only three recipes have been transcribed in the preliminary report.[39] So it is hard to draw definitive conclusions as yet, but it is quite likely that the format, and possibly even the contents, of the two texts recorded in the Han imperial library were modeled on these newly discovered materials.

We can only hope that future archaeological discoveries will re-

---

[35] Paul U. Unschuld, *Medicine in China: A History of Pharmaceutics* (Berkeley: University of California Press, 1986), 16.

[36] Donald Harper, trans., *Early Chinese Medical Literature: The Mawangdui Medical Manuscripts* (London: Kegan Paul International, 1998).

[37] Unschuld, *Medicine in China: A History of Pharmaceutics*, 15-16.

[38] Guo Weimin 郭偉民, "Yuanling hou Wu Yang mu fajue he zhujian zhengli gaikuang" 沅陵侯吳陽墓發掘和竹簡整理概況 (Paper Presented at the International Conference on Recently Discovered Chinese Manuscripts, Beijing University, August 19-22, 2000).

[39] Hunan sheng wenwu kaogu yanjiusuo 湖南省文物考古研究所, Huaibei shi wenwu chu 淮北市文物處, and Yuanling xian bowu guan 沅陵縣博物館, "Yuanling Huxishan yihao Han mu fajue jianbao" 沅陵虎溪山一號漢墓發掘簡報, *Wenwu* 文物 1 (2003): 36-55.

veal more material related to the early stages of this tradition of pharmacopeia for women, but perhaps this is merely wishful thinking. For reasons related to funeral ritual practices, social status, and ideology, it was not usual for women to have been buried with texts, as men were. One of the few exceptions discovered to date is the late western Han tomb at Yinwan 尹灣, Lianyungang 連雲港, Jiangsu, in February 1993, where a married couple was buried together with a large corpus of textual material.[40] A copy of the *Lienü zhuan* is itemized on a tablet listing the contents of the tomb, but most regrettably was not found among the remains.[41] If it had, it would have been a remarkable find, for the author Liu Xiang was probably still alive when the couple was buried. So this newly composed work was probably the wife's favorite reading material. Nevertheless, the evidence quoted above suggests that, even if not theorized, women's bodies must have been considered in some ways different from men's in pre-Han and Han times.[42]

[40] Lianyungang shi bowu guan 連雲港市博物館, Zhongguo shehui kexue yuan jianbo yanjiu zhongxin 中國社會科學院簡帛研究中心, Donghai bowu guan 東海博物館, and Zhongguo wenwu yanjiu suo 中國文物研究所, eds., *Yinwan Han mu jiandu* 尹灣漢墓簡牘 (Beijing: Zhonghua shuju, 1997). Liu Hongshi 劉洪石, "Qiance chutan" 遣冊初探, in Lianyungang shi bowu guan and Zhongguo wenwu yanjiu suo, eds., *Yinwan Han mu jiandu zonglun* 尹灣漢墓簡牘綜論, 123, reads *zhuan* 傳 as *fu* 傅, but says that this is probably the *Lienü zhuan*. It was not the only text mentioned in the tomb inventory that was not found in the tomb.

[41] See Lianyungang shi bowu guan, et al., *Yinwan Han mu jiandu* , tablet 13 recto, 131.

[42] The *Lingshu* 靈樞, *juan* 10, section 65, contains a short essay in which the Yellow Emperor asks his minister Qi Bo 歧伯 why women do not have hair on their face and whether they lack Blood and *qi*. Qi Bo explains that women have an excess of *qi* and an insufficiency of Blood at birth, so that Blood is not able to rise up the penetrating and conception vessels to their lips with the result that facial hair does not grow. See Wu Jing-Nuan, trans., *Ling Shu or The Spiritual Pivot* (Washington, D.C.: Taoist Center, 1993), 213-14. This essay has nothing to do with the ostensible subject of the section *Wuyin wuwei* 五音五味 (The five tones and the five flavors), so it is probably a later composition inserted into the text. Its precise dating I leave to others, although Wang claims the text of the entire *Lingshu* dates from Warring States times, which is very unlikely. Ma Dazheng, *Zhongguo fuchanke fazhan shi*, 24-29, assumes that the *Huangdi neijing*, the *Suwen*, and the *Lingshu* are all texts dating from Warring States times, and so uses quotations from all these canonical sources as evidence for the way women's bodies were conceived and the way women's illnesses were treated using the medicine of systematic correspondence. This assumption is likewise erroneous.

Medicine for Women in the Early Empire and Period of Division

Zhang Ji 張機 (Zhang Zhongjing 張仲景) of the late second century CE, the reputed author of the famous *Shanghan lun* 傷寒論 (Treatise on Cold-induced bodily injuries), included a section on women's illnesses in his *Jingui yuhan yaolüe* 金櫃玉函要略 (Survey of the most important elements from the golden chest and jade casket). Originally this essay may have included twenty-six or thirty-six disorders. Thirty-six would accord with Han numerology, six being even and a *yin* number and the number that correlates with water in the Five Phase philosophical system.[43] Here we find that Zhang considers medical problems for women who are pregnant up to the seventh month and then postpartum. This suggests that the final stages of pregnancy and the birth process itself was not a domain that male doctors intervened in, leaving the care of the mother in the hands of midwives and other expert females, including female shamans and older women of the household. Zhang does not recommend acupuncture, or needling, as an appropriate therapy for women's disorders, rather all his prescriptions, or at least those that have survived, are based on combinations of herbal drugs, providing further support to the idea that the prescriptions in the book in the Han bibliography were also so constituted.[44] Indeed, the slightly later *Maijing* 脈經 (Vessel canon) by the Jin dynasty doctor Wang Shuhe 王叔和 (256 or 265-316), who relies heavily on Zhang Ji, states specifically that a pregnant woman should not be needled, for if she is, she will lose the baby.[45] Huangfu Mi 皇甫謐 (215-82), in his *Zhenjiu jiayi jing* 鍼灸甲乙經 (The A and B canon of needling and moxibustion) recommends needling only when it is clear that the baby has died *in utero*,[46] and this practice was endorsed by many later gyne-

---

[43] Zhang Ji, *Jingui yaolue lunzhu* 金櫃要略論注, *Siku quanshu zhenben siji* 四庫全書珍本四集, 136.20-22. The number 26 appears on 22.8b. See also Zhang Jianrong 張建榮, *Jingui furen sanshiliu bing* 金櫃婦人三十六病 (Beijing: Renmin weisheng chubanshe, 2001).

[44] Wei Zheng 魏徵, ed., *Suishu* 隋書, "Jingji zhi" 經籍志 (Beijing: Zhonghua shuju 1973), *ce* 4, 34.1045, records a book of Zhang's recipes for women, the *Zhang Zhongjing liao furen fang* 張仲景療婦人方 (Zhang Zhongjing's methods of treating women) in two *juan*, but it is no longer extant, so it is not clear whether this was a work actually composed by Zhang or merely attributed to him in later times.

[45] *Maijing*, in Zhongguo yixue dacheng zhengli weiyuan hui 中國醫學大成整理委員會, ed., *Zhongguo yixue dacheng* 中國醫學大成, vol. 3 (Beijing: Zhongguo Zhongyiyao chubanshe, 1997), 9.83.

[46] Zhang Canxia and Xu Guoqian 徐國仟, chief eds., *Zhenjiu jiayi jing jiaozhu*

cological specialists, such as the Song expert Qi Zhongfu 齊仲甫 (1195-1224).[47]

It is fascinating to note that Zhang also includes one section on a problem that he may have encountered in a woman during or shortly after menopause, where he discusses the case of a fifty-year-old woman suffering from menstrual flow lasting several weeks, "hot flashes" at night, a sense of fullness and anxiousness in the belly, heat in the palms of the hands, and dry lips. His diagnosis of the problem is that extravasated Blood from a partial pregnancy from her child-bearing years has collected in the lower abdomen and not been expelled from the body. He proposed to treat the problem with a "soup for warming the circulation tracts," the dispensing of soups being his preferred method of treatment for postpartum disorders.

A second important point to note in Zhang Ji's work is that when he discusses the general origin of women's disorders, he does not gender them.[48] Rather he states that they arise from depletion as a result of an accumulation of Cold inhibiting the flow of *qi* through the circulation tracts, although he also pays considerable attention to the emotions as factors causing illness in women.[49] I will argue later that the gendering of medicine appears only in the Sui and Tang periods in the sixth and seventh centuries.

Turning back to the history of drugs, what Unschuld says about the Chinese pharmacopeia or *bencao* 本草 tradition as a whole seems to be true, that it was not comprehensively theorized and incorporated into the medicine of systematic correspondence until the Song dynasty.[50] In this way, it resembles gynecology in Furth's interpretation. Yet it is clear that as early as the middle of the Han dynasty, at the turn of the millennium, there had developed a coherent tradition in which certain formulae and certain drugs were considered appropriate to treat women's diseases and medical conditions.

鍼灸甲乙經校注 (Beijing: Renmin weisheng chubanshe, 1996), 2.1890-1904. Tana, *Ishinpo*, 3, 22.867-72, "Renfu maitu yue jinfa diyi" 妊婦脈圖月禁法第一, also forbids needling when a woman is pregnant.

47 *Chanbao zalu* 產寶雜錄, late Ming Chongzhen 崇禎 *keben* edition preserved in the Zhongguo kexueyuan tushuguan 中國科學院圖書館, *Xuxiu Siku quanshu*, ed., vol. 1007 (Shanghai: Shanghai guji chubanshe, 1997), 10a-b, 185.

48 Zhang Ji, *Jingui yaolue lunzhu*, 22.8a.

49 Lin Lijia 林立佳, "Zhongjing fuke bing bianzheng ji fangyao tedian fenxi" 仲景婦科病辨證及方藥特點分析, in Wang Qingguo 王慶國, ed., *Zhongjing xueshu yanjiu* 仲景學術研究 (Beijing: Xueyuan chubanshe, 2003), 83-85.

50 Unschuld, *Medicine in China: A History of Pharmaceutics*, 85-127.

For example, the canonical text of the pharmacopeia, the *Shen Nong bencao jing* of the early Eastern Han dynasty,[51] lists ninety types of drugs, including vegetable, animal, and mineral, used to treat women's diseases.[52] Among them is the insect *shufu* 鼠婦 (literally, "mouse woman"), some kind of wood louse or silverfish that lived beneath houses, as being particularly useful in treating retention of urine and blocked menses as well as dispersing blockages of Blood among other conditions.[53] It is possible that this insect was considered efficacious because its intrinsic therapeutic properties had been discovered by chance, or because being close to the earth, which was associated with *yin* in the Han cosmological system, and living beneath houses, where women were located in the Confucian ideological system, they were considered particularly appropriate for use in treating women's health problems. Other drugs are unsystematically recorded as having a particular importance for women. For example, at least two drugs are said in the *Shanhaijing* 山海經 to help women produce children, whereas one found on Mount Bozhong 嶓冢之山 destroys the ability to have children, though this drug could be for both men and women.[54]

---

[51] For a comprehensive discussion of the problems of dating this text, see Wang Jiakui 王家葵 and Zhang Ruixian 張瑞賢, *Shen Nong Bencao jing yanjiu* 神農本草經研究 (Beijing: Beijing kexue jishu chubanshe, 2001), 13-66.

[52] By the time of Tao Hongjing 陶弘景 (456-536), drugs were categorized according to a cosmological system based on the triad Heaven, Man, and Earth. The upper class contained the "rulers," consisting of 120 kinds of drugs; the middle class was called "ministers," also 120 in number; and the lower class contained 125. Thus the combined total was 365, to correspond with the number of degrees in the heavens and the number of days in a year (Unschuld, *Medicine in China: A History of Pharmaceutics*, 19). It was the drugs of the lowest grade, corresponding to Earth, that actually controlled the treatment of disease. Drugs were also classified into categories of *yin* and *yang* and the Five Flavors, with four kinds of *qi*, relationships they had with each other, modeled on human relationships—such as elder brother-younger brother, mother-child and so on—, and whether the drugs continued another's efficacy, feared each other, hated each other, opposed each other, or killed each other. Emotions also had to be taken into consideration when prescribing drugs. See *Lingshu jing* in Ren Jiyu, ed., *Zhongguo kexue jishu dianji tonghui*, "Yixue," section 63, 1.406-07, which contains a discourse on how the Five Flavors act on the various internal organs.

[53] *Shen Nong bencao jing* 神農本草經 in Cao Bingzhang 曹炳章, ed., *Zhongguo yixue dacheng* 中國醫學大成 (Changsha: Yuelu shushe, 1990), vol. 2, "Xiajing" 下經, 44; Ren Jiyu, ed. *Zhongguo kexue jishu dianji tonghui*, "Yixue juan," vol. 1, 3.35a, 591.

[54] Yuan Ke 袁珂, ed., *Shanhaijing jiaozhu* 山海經校注, "Xishan jing" 西山經, *juan* 3 (Shanghai: Shanghai guji chubanshe, 1980), 28.

In the period between the Han and the late Tang (third to tenth centuries), many texts were written either exclusively on women's medicine or on childbirth, or incorporated sections on both, but most of them have been lost. Nevertheless, it is clear that knowledge about the female body and the illnesses that it could succumb to during pregnancy developed quite rapidly. Huangfu Mi devotes a section of his third-century work on acupuncture to the *Furen zabing* 婦人雜病 (Various illnesses of women) and provides a lengthy list of illnesses that can be identified through the vessel-pulses (*mai* 脈), starting with the observation that you can tell whether a woman is pregnant when her body (*shen* 身) is ill or in disorder (*bing* 病) but her vessel-pulses reveal no presence of heteropathy (*xie* 邪).[55] His slightly junior contemporary, the renowned southern Daoist and alchemist Ge Hong 葛洪 (Baopuzi 抱樸子) (284-364), evidently compiled a significant number of recipes to treat women's illnesses, many of which have been preserved by the Japanese scholar Tana Yasuyori, who culled a huge range of Chinese medical works and copied them into his compendium *Ishinpo* (completed in 982, just after the beginning of the Song dynasty in China in 960).[56] These recipes would have been categorized in the developing *bencao* pharmacopeia tradition. They range from recipes to treat pain in the Heart during pregnancy (with a concoction derived from boiled green bamboo skin),[57] blood in the urine (with a concoction derived from boiled plantain, *cheqiancao* 車前草, *Plantago major*),[58] and menorrhagia (*loubao* 漏胞) (with five *liang* 兩 of *ajiao* 阿膠 [ass-hide glue] mixed with five *liang* of dried *Rehmannia glutinosa*, *dihuang* 地黃, boiled in five *sheng* of wine reduced to one and a half *sheng*, drunk warm in two portions before eating);[59] to prevent a fetus from spontaneously aborting when the mother is ill (take mud from the bottom of the well and smear

[55] For the development of vessel theory in the Han, see Elisabeth Hsu, "Pulse Diagnostics in the Western Han: How *Mai* and *Qi* Determine *Bing*," in Elisabeth Hsu, ed., *Innovation in Chinese Medicine* (Cambridge: Cambridge University Press, 2001), 51-91.

[56] A very large number of the texts Tana quoted from were subsequently lost in China, and Tana's own book was retrieved from oblivion in Japan only in the early twentieth century. Some chapters of Tana's work have been translated by Howard S. Levy and Akira Ishihara, *The Tao of Sex: The Essence of Medical Prescriptions (Ishimpō)* (Lower Lake, Calif.: Integral Publishing, 1989).

[57] *Ishinpo*, 3, 22.883.

[58] *Ishinpo*, 3, 21.861.

[59] *Ishinpo*, 3, 22.880.

it three inches below the Heart, a magical operation);[60] and to treat postpartum problems such as failure to expel "bad blood" (masticate three *jin* 斤 of fresh ginger, boil it in one *dou* 斗 of water, reduce to three *sheng*, divide into three portions, and drink).[61]

In chapters 21 to 24 of the *Ishinpo,* devoted to medicine for women, twenty-four out of the forty-eight works that Tana quotes from have as their titles "Prescriptions of such-and such," clearly marking them as belonging to the pharmacopeia tradition, and one of which, the *Qipo fang* 耆婆方 (Prescriptions of Jīvaka), undoubtedly was a Buddhist work as its name derives from a disciple of the Buddha famed for his medical skill, which showed immediately after his birth. He was the son of King Bimbisāra and his concubine Āmrapālī. From this evidence, we can see that prescriptions for women were an integral component of the expanding *bencao* tradition in the centuries following the Han.

How, then, were the works relating to medicine for women and for birthing (midwifery, in Furth's terminology) categorized by the imperial bibliographers? In the catalogue preserved in the history of the Sui dynasty (581-618), we find that birthing manuals are placed in the *Wu xing* 五行 (Five Phase) section, along with numerous types of divination and other manuals, including those for marriage. This section contains the names of eight titles relating to birthing. They are:

Chanru shu 產乳書	(Book on birth and nursing) (2 scrolls)
Chanjing 產經	(Birth canon) (1 scroll)
Tui chanfu heshi chanfa 推產婦何時產法	(Methods for determining the time for parturient mothers to give birth) (1 scroll) by Wang Chen 王琛
Tui chanfa 推產法	(Methods for determining birth) (1 scroll)
Zachan shu 雜產書	(Book of various [matters related to] giving birth) (6 scrolls)
Shengchan fuyi 生產符儀	(Rituals[?] and talismans for giving birth) (1 scroll)
Chantu 產圖	(Birth charts) (2 scrolls)[62]
Zachan tu 雜產圖	(Various charts for giving birth) (4 scrolls)

[60] *Ishinpō*, 3, 22.890.

[61] *Ishinpō*, 3, 23.918.

[62] This text may have been incorporated in the work with the same title by the Tang doctor Cui Zhiti 崔知悌, recorded in the *Jiu Tangshu* 舊唐書 (Beijing: Zhonghua shuju, 1975), 47.2042. Wang Tao 王燾 (fl. ninth century), *Waitai miyao fang* 外台秘要方, in Gao Wenzhu 高文鑄, ed., *Lidai zhongyi mingzhu wenku* 歷代中

Virtually all of these texts are now lost, and we therefore know very little about their contents. However, the *Chanjing* (Birth canon) was composed by the Northern and Southern Dynasties or Sui doctor De Zhenchang 德貞常 who also wrote a work in the pharmacopeia tradition, *De Zhenchang fang* 德貞常方 (De Zhenchang's recipes). From the extensive quotations in the *Ishinpo*, it is evident that not only did De include detailed ritual procedures, hemerological (choosing the right day) prescriptions, guidelines for physiognomizing the newborn infant, and other techniques, which would certainly qualify the text to be categorized in the "Five Phase" section, but he also added long sections on the relations between all the vessel-pulses and the growing fetus, which would normally be associated with acupuncture theory and proper "medicine," and recommendations for the treatment of the expectant mother with pharmaceutical drugs, which would be normally included in the pharmacopeia (*bencao*) category. It must indeed have been a "canon" of all knowledge drawn from many traditions that later bibliographers liked to keep separate. It could have been categorized differently by the Sui imperial librarians. However, integrating ritual and hemerology with medical prescriptions was a feature of later Song birthing manuals and texts on women's medicine, as we will see below, and as Furth has noted.[63] The other texts in the Sui bibliography "Five Phase" section given above, judging from their titles, were most likely concerned primarily with ritual procedures and hemerological considerations involved in childbirth and were thus appropriately categorized in the *Suishu* 隋書. I will discuss below some examples of similar practices and rituals that were probably described in those texts.

醫名著文庫 (Beijing: Huaxia chubanshe, 1993), quotes more than four hundred times from Cui's lost work, *Cuishi zuanyao fang* 崔氏纂要方, and it would appear, according to Gao Wenzhu, "*Waitai miyao fang* yinyong shumu wenxian kaolue" 外臺秘要方引用書目文獻考略, in *Waitai miyao fang*, 1003-04, that his "Birth Chart" was included in chapter 10A of his larger work. Most interestingly, Gao notes that in his preface to the chapter on "Bone-steaming" 骨蒸, which also was transmitted as a separate work, the *Guzheng bingjiu fang* 骨蒸病灸方, preserved in its entirety in chapter 13 of the *Waitai miyao fang*, 233-34, Cui posits that for men suffering from "Bone-steaming" the "*jia-qi*" is the "root" 丈夫以瘕氣爲根, whereas in women it is the "Blood-*qi*" that is fundamental 婦人以血氣爲本. It would be very worthwhile, in my opinion, to trace the development of the notion of "Blood" as fundamental in women through such lost Tang texts as Cui's in order to excavate the immediate prehistory of the notion that became fundamental to the fully fledged gynecology in the Song that Furth has described.

[63] Furth, *A Flourishing Yin*, 306.

Finally, in the section of "medical recipes" ("Yi fang" 醫方) in the Sui bibliography are recorded several works related to medicine for women that have also been lost. They are the anonymous "The Yellow Emperor's plain questions about girls and fetuses[?]" (*Huangdi Suwen nütai* 黃帝素問女胎);[64] "Zhang Zhongjing's methods for treating women," mentioned above;[65] "Various recipes for treating postpartum women" (*Liao furen chanhou zafang* 療婦人產後雜方) in three chapters and "The Yellow Emperor's canon on nourishing the fetus" (*Huangdi yangtai jing* 黃帝養胎經) in one chapter;[66] and "Xu Wenbo's cures for abdominal masses in women" (*Xu Wenbo liao furen jia* 徐文伯療婦人瘕).[67] These presumably were Six Dynasties works in the *bencao* tradition, but their contents cannot be recovered.[68] Two similar works were recorded in the bibliography section of *Jiu Tangshu* 舊唐書, called simply *Furen fang* 婦人方 (Recipes for women); both of these are anonymous and contained ten and twenty chapters, respectively.[69] Again, we cannot recover the contents and nature of their recipes, as they have been lost without trace, although quite possibly later writers on medicine drew on them. Thus there were a number of texts written exclusively on the subject of medicine for women by the beginning of the seventh century, but imperial bibliographers did not categorize them all together. There were also a large number of texts in the *bencao* tradition that included sections on treating women's diseases and problems. But was there a clear tradition of gynecology?

To round out the discussion of medicine for women in the Period of Division, I would like to say a few words about a hitherto neglected technology related to the *bencao* tradition, the tradition of unguents and fragrances. But before I do so, I want to note that the earliest Chinese text devoted exclusively to women's medicine that survives in its entirety is the *Jingxiao chanbao* 經效產寶 by the late Tang doctor Zan Yin 昝殷.[70] This work does not include ritual

---

[64] *Suishu* 34.1043.

[65] See the discussion at the beginning of the section "Medicine for Women in the Early Empire and Period of Division" above and n. 44.

[66] *Suishu* 34.1047.

[67] *Suishu* 34.1045.

[68] I shall discuss below the *Xiaopin fang* 小品方, an influential *bencao* work that we know from surviving fragments contained a section of prescriptions for parturient women.

[69] *Jiu Tangshu*, 47.2050.

[70] The three editions that I have examined are the Guangxu year 7 (1881)

or esoteric practices, but only records a wide range of prescriptions drawn from Zan's own experience and from earlier works dating from the Six Dynasties, Sui, and Tang times. Zan also wrote a book, originally in three chapters, called the *Shiyi xinjian* 食醫心鑒 in the food subcategory of the *bencao* tradition. Parts of this latter work were preserved in a Korean medical compendium.[71] What survives of the latter text's section concerning medicine for women consists of an introductory preface followed by twelve recipes for pregnant women, one recipe for immediately after delivery, and twenty recipes for problems arising later after birth. For example, he recommends treating morning sickness when a pregnant woman finds it hard to eat with a kind of soup noodle (*suobing* 索餅) flavored with mutton or goat's meat, this kind of noodle, without the mutton, being favored by Zhang Ji in the Han for treating a person suffering from Cold damage.

Fragrances and Unguents

The history of unguents and fragrances is a little-explored aspect of the *bencao* tradition of women's medicine.[72] The great early Tang

reprint of the Song dynasty *keben* edition held in the Shanghai cishu chubanshe tushuguan (*Xuxiu Siku quanshu* ed. [Shanghai: Shanghai guji chubanshe, ca. 1997]) 1006.653-92; Wang Zhenrui 王振瑞, Wang Yantian 王彥田, and Niu Bingzhan 牛兵占, eds., in *Zhongyi fuke mingzhu jicheng* 中醫婦科名著集成 (*Lidai Zhongyi mingzhu wenku*, ed.) with a supplement by Zhou Ting 周頲, *Jingxiao chanbao xubian* 經效產寶續編 (Beijing: Huaxia chubanshe, 1997), 1-26; and Zhang Nianshun 張年順, et al., eds., *Zhongguo yixue dacheng*, 7.187-218.

71 Zhu Danian 朱大年, et al., eds., *Lidai bencao jinghua congshu* 歷代本草精華叢書 (Shanghai: Shanghai yiyao daxue chubanshe, 1994), 1.24b-29a. The Korean medical text is the *Yifang leiju* 醫方類聚 (Medical recipes collected by category).

72 Wang Tao, *Waitai miyao fang*, has thirty-four subheadings, with a total of 225 recipes for various unguents, fragrances, hair shampoos, detergents for clothes, and so on, drawn from previous works, such as those composed by Sun Simo, in Chapter 32 of his book, 622-45. The most extensive compendium of descriptions of fragrances, as far as I am aware, is the Song scholar Chen Jing's 陳景 *Chenshi Xiangpu* 陳氏香譜 (*Siku quanshu zhenben*, ed., *Siji*, vol. 194) (Taibei: Wuling chubanshe, 1969) in four chapters. For a brief review of different types of make-up in the Tang, see Charles Benn, *China's Golden Age: Everyday Life in the Tang Dynasty* (Oxford: Oxford University Press, 2002), 107-09, and Edward H. Schafer, "The Early History of Lead Pigments and Cosmetics in China," *T'oung Pao* 44 (1956):413-38. For a compendium of anecdotes about many varieties of women's make-up and clothes through the centuries, see Tian Mai 田霢, *Zhuang shi* 妝史, in *Beijing tushuguan cang guji zhenben congkan* (Beijing: Shumu wenxian chubanshe, 1988), 70.763-823.

doctor, ophthalmologist, and alchemist Sun Simo, in his *Qianjin yifang* 千金翼方 (Supplementary prescriptions worth a thousand gold pieces), in addition to detailing prescriptions for various women's illnesses also provides recipes for fragrances that she can use on her own body and for her clothes. For example, one recipe for scenting the body reads:

> Licorice, five *fen*, roasted, hemlock parsley (*Conioselinum univittatum*), 1 *liang*, and *Angelica anomala*, three *fen*. These three ingredients are ground together and sifted into a powder and a *fangcun* 方寸 spoonful is to be drunk three times a day. In thirty days the mouth is scented and in forty days the body is scented.[73]
>
> 甘草 伍分炙芎藭壹兩白芷參分右參味擣篩爲散以飲服方寸匕日三服三十日口香四十日身香

Another recipe calls for the combining of one *liang* each of three ingredients, the seeds of a gourd (*guazi* 瓜子), the root and white bark of pine, and large jujubes, a *fangcun* spoonful of the powder to be drunk in wine twice a day. In a hundred days both the woman's clothes and coverings will be fragrant.

A combination of similar ingredients is used in a prescription to counter the effects of premature aging and what sounds, possibly, like a form of Alzheimer's disease combined with other troubles.[74] The symptoms of this condition are given as the hair prematurely turning white, depletion and fatigue of the brain and the body, emptiness and exhaustion in the stomach, unbalanced *qi*, all the *zang* 臟 organs depleted and cut off, and the Blood and *qi* insufficient. These conditions result in the hair turning prematurely white. Then thinking about the hair brings on worry and anxiety, induces shortsightedness, Wind and tears are emitted, and the hands and feet are troubled by heat/fever; the woman is confused, forgetful, and makes mistakes, and has diarrhea for years on end. If the prescription is taken for a year, it has a great effect. The prescription is one *sheng* of gourd seeds (*guazi*), *Angelica anomala* (*baizhi*) without the epidermis, two *liang* each of *Angelica polymorpha* (*danggui*), hemlock parsley (*xiongqiong*), and licorice (*gancao*). (Another recipe adds two *liang* of pine nuts). These five ingredients are ground and sifted into a powder, and one *fangcun* spoonful is taken three times a day; it can

---

[73] Sun Simo, *Qianjin yifang* (Supplementary prescriptions worth a thousand gold pieces) (Taibei: Ziyou chubanshe, 1995), 5.69b.

[74] Sun Simo, *Qianjin yifang*, *juan* 5, 71b.

also be consumed with wine, bean sauce, or soup. This is known as *guazi san* 瓜子散, gourd seed powder.

Sun seems to have been drawing on texts such as the one discovered among the Dunhuang hoard at the beginning of the twentieth century belonging to the Buddhist monastery complex in the Gobi Desert at the far northwestern end of the Gansu corridor, and now held in the British Library as Stein manuscript 4329 and given the title *Meirong fangshu* 美容方書 (Book of recipes for a beautiful complexion). The surviving forty-eight-line fragment details twelve different recipes, using up to twenty-one different vegetable and mineral ingredients for treating bad breath, fragrancing clothes, and concocting facial washes, creams and unguents, and hair shampoos.[75] There can be no doubt that these formularies were conceived of as medical as well as ritual in nature and of particular value for women, for many of the ingredients were believed to have properties that expelled poison and stimulated the Blood. Although both males and females had Blood and *qi*, later on, in the Southern Song, Blood was prioritized and considered the primary constituent of females that distinguished the female from the male body. Blood had to be regulated and it is to this rise in Song doctors' concerns with female Blood that Furth largely attributes the gendering of medicine in that time period. She quotes Yang Shiying 楊士瀛 (thirteenth century) as writing:

> Males and females both have Blood and *qi*, yet people say that in women Blood is fundamental. Why? Because their Blood is in ascendancy over *qi*; it is stored in the Liver system, flows through the womb and is ruled by the Heart system; it ascends to become breast milk, descends to become menses, unites with semen to make the embryo.
> 男女均有此血氣,人皆曰婦人以血爲本, 何耶?蓋其血勝於氣耳. 血藏於肝, 流注子臟而主其血者在心上爲乳汁下爲月水合精而爲胞胎 ...[76]

I will consider the question of Blood in pre-Song medicine later on. Here I want to emphasize that from early times a beautiful face was

---

[75] Cong Chunyu 叢春雨, ed., *Dunhuang Zhongyiyao quanshu* 敦煌中醫藥全書, (Complete book of Chinese medicine and drugs from Dunhuang) (Beijing: Zhongyi guji chubanshe, 1994), 641-44. See also his essay "Dunhuang yishu zhong fuke guyi fang de xueshu tedian" 敦煌遺書中婦科古醫方的學術特點, in *Dunhuang Zhongyiyao jingcui fawei* 敦煌中醫藥精萃發微 (Beijing: Zhongyi guji chubanshe, 2000), 358-61.

[76] Furth, *A Flourishing Yin*, 73, quoting Ma Dazheng, *Zhongguo fuchanke fazhan shi*, 151. Furth does not translate the entire passage taken from Yang's *Renzhai zhizhi fanglun* 仁齋直指方論.

considered to be reflective of good inner moral qualities and was one of the primary sites that revealed a person's fate. The art of physiognomy, of course, was focused on interpreting external features that were indicative of life span, good or bad fortune, wealth, rank, moral condition, and personality.[77] At the same time, as Angela Zito has pointed out,

> For the Chinese medical body, boundaries between interior and exterior are conceived dynamically as the point of interface where internal and external processes engage, and this changes according to the point of view or function.[78]

So the face was conceived of not just in aesthetic terms (as pretty, for example), but as the revelatory site where the person expressed herself to the world and received in turn its influences. With respect to external influences, from the medical point of view, we find the Sui doctor Chao Yuanfang 巢元方 (fl. 605-15), in his vast compendium compiled by imperial order, thinking that black facial spots or freckles on a woman had three possible origins: either a blockage of *qi* absorbed as water in the *zang* and *fu* internal organs (*tanyin* 痰飲), or that the face had suffered from an attack of heteropathic Wind, or that the woman's Blood and *qi* had become unbalanced. If the eruption of the spots had resulted from an attack of Wind, then he believed it could be treated externally, but if it was the result of an internal organic problem, then it had to be treated internally.[79] Thus trouble with the face could be symptomatic of a dangerous medical condition that called for immediate treatment.

Finally, I should note the ritual importance of washing the hair in early China. Essentially, the hair was conceived of as a condensed symbol of the self. If physical and ritual purity was to be achieved, a purity that enabled one to participate in sacred acts, such as sacrificing to the ancestors or the spirits, carrying out one's official duties as a bureaucrat, paying a formal visit to someone higher in the social or bureaucratic hierarchy, or especially paying respects to the

---

[77] Richard J. Smith, *Fortune-Tellers and Philosophers: Divination in Traditional Chinese Society* (Boulder: Westview Press, 1991), 173-219.

[78] Angela Zito, "Silk and Skin: Significant Boundaries," in Angela Zito and Tani E. Barlow eds., *Body, Subject and Power in China* (Chicago: University of Chicago Press, 1994), 110.

[79] Quoted in the *Ishinpo*, 3, 21.842-43. For symptoms and treatment of the condition of *tanyin*, see Chao Yuanfang, "Zhubing yuanhou lun jiaozhu" 諸病源候論校注, in Ding Guangdi 丁光迪, ed. (Beijing: Renmin weisheng chubanshe, 1996), 1.598-608.

emperor, it was necessary to wash one's hair in advance and to desist from sexual relations and from consuming meat.[80] The hair was a site significative of ritual purity or pollution. We should therefore interpret the recipes used for fragrancing the clothes, washing the hair, and making up the face as much more than efforts by women to make themselves attractive to their spouses. They may have been that, but they were also guarding themselves against heteropathic Wind and trying to ensure that their Blood and *qi* were balanced and that they were able to function as partners of their husbands in performing ritual sacrifices.

The Beginnings of the Gendering of Medicine

As the nineteen-chapter Han dynasty work *Prescriptions for Women and Children* mentioned above is no longer extant, it is not possible to say precisely how specific prescriptions for women evolved over the centuries from the Han to the Song, nor how knowledge about women's bodies was conceptualized in the early empire. The likelihood is, however, that more drugs in a wider variety of combinations were recommended for a greater variety of syndromes, as pharmacological and medical knowledge increased rather than suffering after the Han the kind of collapse in knowledge that the West experienced after the fall of the Roman Empire. It is also clear that a number of texts over the centuries took up the challenge of recommending formulas for treating sick women and providing recommendations for women's pregnancy and childbirth. As discussed above, a number of texts concerned with medicine for women are recorded in the Sui dynasty imperial bibliography, together with some "birth charts" (*chantu*).[81] Lee Jen-der would seem to be correct in suggesting that there was a significant change in medical thinking in about the seventh century.[82] While I cannot accept her view that it was only then

---

[80] Robin D. S. Yates, "Purity and Pollution in Early China," *Zhongguo kaoguxue yu lishixue zhenghe yanjiu* 中國考古學與歷史學整合研究 (Integrated Studies of Chinese Archaeology and History, Symposium Series of the Institute of History and Philology, Academia Sinica, No. 4, Taipei, 1997), 479-536.

[81] See the discussion of the texts recorded in the bibliography of the *Suishu* above.

[82] Li Zhende, "Han Tang zhijian qiuzi yifang shitan" and "Han Tang zhijian yishu zhong de shangchan zhi dao."

that an independent genre of medical writing of "recipes for women" developed, for the evidence seems strong that it had existed ever since the Han or even earlier, as I have shown, yet she is correct to point out that it was in the Sui and early Tang that writers began to theorize about the reasons for the differences between therapies for men and for women. It was then that Chinese medicine really began to be gendered and gender differences between male and female bodies began to be accentuated.

This development is indicated in a famous passage by Sun Simo's *Beiji qianjin yaofang* 備急千金要方 (Essential prescriptions worth a thousand gold pieces) that became, as Furth observes,[83] the foundation stone for the development of gynecology in the Song. The essay was frequently quoted by later writers on women's disorders, either in part or in whole. Tana abstracts two passages from it at the beginning of his own section on medicine for women starting with Chapter 21.1, "Furen zhubing suoyou" 婦人諸病所由 (The origin of all illnesses in women):

> The *Qianjin fang* states: The Treatise states: "Now the reason why women have different prescriptions is because of the difference that their Blood and *qi* are not harmonized, they become pregnant and give birth to children, and suffer from bleeding [from the uterus]. For this reason women's illnesses are ten times more difficult to cure than men's ... With respect to illnesses deriving from the *qi* of the four seasons and damage from deficiency and repletion, Cold or Heat, they are the same as their husbands'. It is only when she suffers from illness when pregnant that she should avoid potent [poisonous] medicines."
>
> It also states: "A woman's desires are more numerous than those of her husband, and if she is affected by illness then it is more serious than in a man. Add to that her compassion and affections, her loves and hatreds, her jealousies and envies, her worries and anger, which are as deep as a solid prison, and she cannot suppress her feelings by herself, and therefore the roots of illnesses are deep and the cures are more difficult to effect. . . . Therefore the attendants of the governess [women in wealthy aristocratic families responsible for looking after the womenfolk in a household] also absolutely must study [presumably these three chapters in Sun Simo's book] and be constantly on guard to check their charges' health."[84]
>
> 千金方云論曰夫婦人所以有別方者以其血氣不調胎妊產生崩傷之異故也所以婦人之病比之男子十倍難療若四時節氣爲病虛實冷熱爲患者與丈夫同也唯懷胎妊挾病者避其毒藥耳

---

[83] *A Flourishing Yin*, 71-72.

[84] Sun Simo, *Beiji qianjin yaofang* (*Siku quanshu* reprint ed.), in Ren Jiyu, ed., *Zhongguo kexue jishu dianji tonghui*, "Yixue," 2.217 (2.1a-2a).

又云女人嗜欲多於丈夫感病則倍於男子加以慈戀愛憎嫉妒懮恚深着堅牢情不自抑所以爲病根深療之難瘥故傅母之徒亦不可不學

The reason Sun Simo points to the emotions as a problem for women is that it was believed that the unregulated emotions of happiness and anger were one of the prime causes of diseases, together with the exogenous factors of wind, rain, cold, heat, and dampness. When these emotions were unregulated, the *zang* organs were damaged, and the resulting illness arose from *yin*. In particular, sadness was believed to damage the Heart and anger the Liver.[85]

In an interesting omission, Tana fails to mention that Sun also quotes the medical canon that women are gathering places for the multitude of *yin* energies and always live in damp locations, thus the Japanese scholar excludes external factors affecting women's health that derived partially from social practices.[86] By this I mean that the inner quarters where women lived and worked were usually located for geomantic reasons in the northern, *yin*, part of a dwelling complex. Tana also omits another paragraph saying that women's dis-

---

[85] *Lingshu jing*, *juan* 10, section 66, Ren Jiyu, ed., *Zhongguo kexue jishu dianji tonghui*, "Yixue" 1, 412-14; Wu Jing-nuan, trans., Lingshu, *216*. See also Zhang Ji's opinions on this matter, in the section "Medicine for Women in the Early Empire and Period of Division" above.

[86] Instead of quoting the whole of Sun Simo's treatise, Tana quotes the fifth-century work *Xiaopin fang*, saying: "In the past, women's illnesses were easy to cure. They married late, their Kidney *qi* was settled, and that was the reason they rarely fell ill and did not suffer very much. Nowadays, they marry early before the root of their Kidneys is settled, and then giving birth damages their Kidneys, and for these reasons today's young married women fall sick and inevitably they are hard to cure. Early marriage and giving birth early, even if no illness ensues, is calamitous" (Gao Wenzhu, 128). The dating of the *Xiaopin fang* is disputed. See Li Zhende, "Han Tang zhijian qiuzi yifang shitan," 301 n. 71. Ma Jixing, "*Yixin fang* zhong de gu yixue wenxian chutan" 醫心方中的古醫學文獻初探, *Nihon igaku zasshi* 日本醫學雜誌 31.3 (1985):326-71 (30-75), thinks it is of Jin date; Ma Dazheng, *Zhongguo fuchanke fazhan shi*, 53, thinks it was composed at the interstices of the two Jin dynasties, that is, the early fourth century; Tang Wanchun 湯萬春, in commenting on Chen Yanzhi 陳延之 in *Xiaopin fang jilu jianzhu* 小品方輯錄箋注 (Anhui: Kexue jishu chubanshe, 1990) thinks it is of the Northern and Southern dynasties period; Ren Xu 任旭, "*Xiaopin fang* canjuan jianjie" 小品方殘卷簡介, *Zhonghua yishi zazhi* 中華醫史雜誌 17.2 (1987):71-73; and Liao Yuqun 廖育群, "Chen Yanzhi yu *Xiaopin fang* yanjiu de xin jinzhan" 陳延之與小品方研究的新進展, *Zhonghua yishi zazhi* 17 (1987):74-75, think that is of the Liu Song dynasty. Lee Jen-der concurs with Ren and Liao's views. See also Liao Yuqun, Fu Fang 傅芳, and Zheng Jinsheng 鄭金生, *Zhongguo kexue jishu shi* 中國科學技術史, "Yixue juan" 醫學卷 (Beijing: Kexue chubanshe, 1998), 218-19, and Yan Shiyun 嚴世芸, chief ed., *Zhongguo yiji tongkao* 中國醫籍通考 (Shanghai: Shanghai Zhongyi xueyuan chubanshe, 1992), 2.2085-86.

eases originate from the onset of their menses at age 14 *sui*. At that age, Sun states, women's

> *Yin qi* overflows and numerous thoughts pass through their Hearts, damaging their five organs on the inside and ruining their facial complexion on the outside. Their monthly courses flow out or are retained within, now early, now late, stagnating and congesting Blood and interrupting the functions of central pathways. The injuries from this cannot be enumerated in words. Internal organs are now Cold, now Hot, now replete, now depleted. Bad Blood within leaks out, and energy channels are used up and drained empty. Sometimes immoderate diet causes damage, sometimes they have sexual intercourse before their [vaginal] itching sores have healed. Sometimes as they relieve themselves at the privy above, Wind from below enters, causing the twelve chronic illnesses. All of this is why women have separate prescriptions.[87]
> 陰氣浮溢百想經心內傷五臟外損姿顏月水去留前後交互瘀血停凝中道斷絕其中傷墮不可具論生熟二臟虛實交錯惡血內漏氣脈損竭或飲食無度損傷非一或瘡痍未愈便合陰陽或便利於懸廁之上風從下入便成十二痼疾所以婦人別立方也

Here Sun is prioritizing the effects of irregular menstrual flow as well as the normal process of menstruation as the cause of women's suffering more diseases than men and therefore needing different prescriptions. This emphasis on Blood, as Furth cogently argues, became the basis for doctors in the Song and later to integrate women's problems within a specific paradigm of diagnosis. At the same time, Sun also attributes women's diseases to another, incompatible, source: their squatting in the toilet makes possible for harmful Wind to enter their lower orifices and thus, although Sun does not say so specifically, cause Cold damage. Sun, in fact, is drawing here on the etiology proposed by Zhang Ji in the Han. Indeed, Sun's older contemporary, Chao Yuanfang, also attributes many of women's medical problems to Cold damage caused by Wind. Unschuld claims that Zhang Ji's "works exerted only marginal influence on medical thought and literature between the Han and Sung [Song] dynasties"[88] and that his ideas were really only rediscovered and developed by doctors of the Song, Jin, and Yuan at which time a "restricted etiology" for disease was adopted.[89] This interpretation does not seem to be true of Zhang's writings on women's health. It is likely, in my opinion, that Zhang's ideas were transmitted in the medical tradition through their influence and role in gynecolo-

---

[87] Sun Simo, *Beiji qianjin yaofang* 2.217 (2.1a-b); translated by Furth, *A Flourishing Yin*, 71, with some amendments.

[88] Unschuld, *Medicine in China: A History of Ideas*, 168.

[89] Unschuld, *Medicine in China: A History of Ideas*, 168.

gy before they were picked up and expanded in the "renaissance" of Zhang Ji's thought from the eleventh through fourteenth centuries. In addition, lying behind Sun's concerns about the dangers of the toilet are beliefs and practices associated with popular religion. I will consider ritual in the birthing process below, but here I just want to point out that toilets were considered to be sites of pollution and locations where dangerous ghosts lay hidden, not only because that was where defecation and urination took place, in other words human excreta or waste, "matter out of place" in Mary Douglas's terminology,[90] were deposited, but also because toilets were where women raised silkworms, notorious for their waste production, and fed pigs. Thus toilets were sites of *yin*, of pollution, and particularly under the control of women. Following geomantic principles, they were always located in the north, *yin*, side of a housing complex.

Reading through Chao Yuanfang and Sun Simo's treatises also reveals another important phenomenon. Acupuncture was only used in very rare circumstances as therapy for pregnant, parturient, or postpartum women. In fact, needling is only used when a woman no longer is producing children, when she can no longer receive sperm,[91] when she has suffered miscarriages, or when there are problems with her menses.[92] Tana observed this feature, quoting the *Qianjin fang* as stating, "Prescription for terminating births: Cauterize one inch above the right ankle three times (*sanzhuang* 三壯), then she will stop."[93] He adds another prescription, "(Take) old cloth made from silkworms one foot (*chi* 尺) square, burn it to powder, and drink it with wine," an act that Chen Yanzhi's fifth-century *Xiaopin fang* (Recipes of small pieces) claimed would terminate pregnancies for the rest of a woman's life.[94] Thus doctors were prepared to re-

---

[90] Mary Douglas, *Purity and Danger: An Analysis of the Concepts of Pollution and Taboo* (London: Ark Paperbacks, 1984), 40.

[91] Sun Simo, *Beiji qianjin yaofang*, 2. 222-223 (2.11b-12a).

[92] Sun Simo, *Beiji qianjin yaofang*, 2.279-80 (5.26a-27a).

[93] Sun Simo, *Beiji qianjin yaofang*, 2.280 (5.27a).

[94] *Ishinpo* 3, 21.863. I have not been able to find this recipe in Gao Wenzhu, ed., *Xiaopin fang* (Beijing: Zhongguo zhongyiyao chubanshe, 1995), 7.128-49. It was quoted at the end of Chapter 34 of Wang Tao's *Waitai miyao fang*, 700, where Gao Wenzhu notes that Sun Simo's *Beiji qianjin yaofang* 2.277 (5.22b) (not quoting from the *Xiaopin* explicitly) reads "old silkworm paper" *canzi guzhi* 蠶子故紙. This is probably a mistake in the transmission of the *Beiji qianjin yaofang* text, as Sun's *Qianjin yifang*, Zhu Bangxian 朱邦賢 and Chen Wenguo 陳文國, eds., *Qianjin yifang jiaozhu* 千金翼方校注 (Shanghai: Shanghai guji chubanshe, 1999), 155, a work that Sun

cord prescriptions that enabled women to escape the constant, and possibly debilitating, repetition of the reproductive cycle, a textual inscription that must have provided relief to innumerable women over the centuries in both China and Japan.[95] I should also note, in the light of this evidence, that acupuncture should not be given an equal place in the list of therapies in the clinical tradition of gynecology, if gynecology is defined as the medicine practiced on women during their reproductive activities. The use of drugs drawn from an extensive pharmacopeia was far more important.

One last comment is relevant here on the use of old silkworm cloth to terminate reproduction. As Francesca Bray has pointed out in her excellent book, the production of cloth was considered to be the work of women par excellence, and it was what tied the woman to her family, her community, and the state, to the latter in the form of taxes.[96] At the same time, women created their own subjectivity throughout their production of cloth. Not only was the cloth they wove a form of currency at least through the Tang dynasty, but that cloth was also taken by them as their dowry in marriage, thus creating status and giving them economic resources separate from those of their husbands. Cloth also represented women's moral virtues. As Bray puts it so cogently, "By spinning and weaving, women produced not only objects of value but also persons of virtue. Learning textile skills inculcated the fundamental female values of diligence, frugality, order and self-discipline."[97] In the case of the old cloth for terminating pregnancy, the woman is taking an object

composed at the end of his life, gives the phrase as *gu canzi bu* 故蠶子布, although the Northern Song edition of the *Beiji qianjin yaofang*, reprinted by the Edo Igaku [Jianghu Yixue 江戶醫學 (1878)], and reprinted in the *Zhongguo yixue dacheng xuji* 中國醫學大成續集 (Shanghai: Shanghai kexue jishu chubanshe, 2000), 3.201, also writes "old paper." The discrepancy might also be explained by Sun changing his mind on this issue in later life.

95 The last section of the gynecology chapter, 34, of the *Waitai miyao fang*, 700, contains three other prescriptions for stopping pregnancies, one of them from Sun Simo, which recommends drinking mercury (*shuiyin* 水銀) that has been boiled for a whole day. Although Sun claims that it is not harmful to humans (that is, the mother), one hopes that not too many women resorted to this poisonous remedy (only women aristocrats would have been able to afford it or have the means to acquire it).

96 Francesca Bray, *Technology and Gender: Fabrics of Power in Late Imperial China* (Berkeley: University of California Press, 1997).

97 Bray, *Technology and Gender*, 189.

of her own labor that symbolized all her productive and reproductive capacity and her moral virtues to subvert and terminate that very productivity and reproductivity. It is an act of powerful agency, one that would initiate a new stage in her life, less subject to the physical demands of her husband.[98] Within the social and religious context of medieval China, of course, it might also have been a liberating act for a woman who was a devout Buddhist, for it would permit her to practice her religion with greater equanimity and with greater adherence to its fundamental precepts, unsoiled by desires that were the fundamental barrier to religious transformation.[99]

---

[98] I am not suggesting here that a woman, as a faithful Buddhist who would not have believed in killing, is engaging in an act that could be interpreted as abortion or willful killing of her unborn fetus; she is merely terminating her ability to produce children. I am, of course, aware that incinerated cloth was used for various purposes in premodern Chinese medicine. In the present instance, I am trying to interpret the medical practices. A further example can be taken from Sun Simo. He suggested one way of stopping blood flowing continuously from a young girl (*tongnü* 童女), probably one who was not yet married, when injured in the vagina by the inappropriate entrance of a male member or other object, was to burn a green-colored cloth together with hair and to smear the ash on the injury with the result that the bleeding would, he thought, immediately stop (*Beiji qianjin yaofang*, Northern Song edition, *Zhongguo yixue dacheng xuji*, 3.210). Here the green color may symbolize spring, youth, and fertility, while the hair may be symbol of the pubic hair and the entire body, but whether there was a connection with the use of a green cloth and hair in other rituals, such as death rituals, awaits further research. On this latter point, in contemporary Cantonese funerals, James L. Watson observed that daughters-in-law wear green cloths over their abdomen "in such a manner as to cover the female reproductive organs" and notes that the green color absorbs death pollution. These cloths are then passed over fire to purify them and used to make the centerpiece of the backstrap of the harnesses for their infants. Further, married daughters rub their hair on the deceased's coffin to absorb the death pollution. Death pollution thus, in Watson's opinion, actually creates fertility. See James L. Watson, "Of Flesh and Bones: The Management of Death Pollution in Cantonese Society," in Maurice Bloch and Jonathan Parry, eds., *Death and the Regeneration of Life* (Cambridge: Cambridge University Press, 1982), 174-75. This is remarked upon by Emily Martin in her "Gender and Ideological Representations of Life and Death," in James L. Watson and Evelyn S. Rawski, eds., *Death Ritual in Late Imperial and Modern China* (Berkeley: University of California Press, 1988), 172. Were the burned green cloth and the hair intended to have the same function, to absorb the pollution of the blood flow from a young woman who should not have been penetrated? It is impossible to know for certain. But I believe it is incumbent on us to try to interpret the cultural meanings of the ingredients and practices we find in early Chinese medicine.

[99] The five fundamental precepts of a Buddhist householder were not harming living creatures, not lying, not engaging in wrong sexual conduct, not stealing, and not drinking intoxicating substances. An additional three were not applying perfume

Ritual and Women's Medicine

Another exceptionally important aspect of gynecology in early imperial times is the role of religious ritual in medicine for women. I mentioned before that women appear in the Han imperial bibliography in two places. The first was in the recipes section discussed above. They also appear in the succeeding section, on "Arts of the Bedchamber."[100] As with the case of the "recipes," none of the eight works in a total of 185 rolls listed is extant, but a good sense of their likely contents has been preserved in the earlier, and probably ancestral, texts found in the tomb at Mawangdui. As these latter texts have been ably translated and commented upon by several scholars, notably Donald Harper,[101] Douglas Wile,[102] and Li Ling and Keith McMahon,[103] among others,[104] I will not discuss these in any detail in the present essay.

Rather, I would like to draw attention to the close relation this genre of esoteric writing on *yangsheng* 養生 (nourishing life), which in the later and post-Han period was developed by Daoists principally to enhance the prospects for longevity for male practitioners, had to medical works providing guidelines for women going through the process of fertilization, pregnancy, delivery, and the experience after birth. Indeed, the last text in the section in the Han bibliog-

---

to the body, not wearing adornments, not watching entertainment or listening to singing; not sitting or lying on a high or wide bed; and not eating at proscribed times. See Kathryn Ann Tsai, *Lives of the Nuns: Biographies of Chinese Buddhist Nuns from the Fourth to the Sixth Centuries* (Honolulu: University of Hawaii Press, 1994), 122 n. 52, and 125 n. 83. Many of the recipes recorded in the gynecological texts suggest that the potion be drunk with alcoholic liquor; it is not unlikely, in my opinion, that a woman who was strictly adhering to the Buddhist vows would not use such potions, preferring the alternatives that did not require her to drink liquor. There is, however, no hard evidence to support such a speculation.

[100] *Hanshu*, 30.1778-79.

[101] Harper, trans., *Early Chinese Medical Literature: The Mawangdui Medical Manuscripts*.

[102] Wile, *The Chinese Sexual Yoga Classics Including Women's Solo Meditation Texts* (Albany: State University of New York Press, 1992).

[103] Li Ling and Keith McMahon, "The Contents and Terminology of the Mawangdui Texts on the Arts of the Bedchamber," *Early China* 17 (1992):145-85.

[104] For a study of a Tang dynasty rhapsody attributed to the younger brother of the famous Tang poet Bo Juyi 白居易 (772-846), Bo Xingjian 白行簡 (776?-826), related to the arts of the bedchamber, see Sumiyo Umekawa, "*Tiandi yinyang jiaohuang dalefu* and the Art of the Bedchamber," in Lo and Cullen, eds., *Medieval Chinese Medicine*, 252-77.

raphy is titled *Sanjia neifang youzi fang* 三家內房有子方 (The three masters' recipes for having children in the bedchamber).[105] Furthermore, Sun Simo, at the end of his treatise on childbirth that I quoted extensively above, recommends that "Masters of Nourishing Life especially must teach boys and girls (perhaps sons and daughters) to study and practice the following three chapters," namely those starting with prescriptions on how to produce a child for childless couples, through pregnancy and birth to postpartum problems (*juan* 2 through 4). Of course, he also intended his audience to include matrons whom he refers to as "attendants of the governess," women in wealthy aristocratic families responsible for looking after the womenfolk in a household. He assumes such older women were literate and able to instruct their charges in the procedures he details, as well as being capable of preparing the complex formulas he provides and of administering the drugs.

We also find that Tana quoted extensively from works in this same Daoist "nourishing life" tradition. These are the *Yangsheng yaoji* 養生要集 (The essential collection on nourishing life) of the Jin dynasty, a work from which Chao Yuanfang also quotes extensively in its sections on gymnastics as a means of curing disease, the *Yangsheng fang* 養生方 (Recipes for nourishing life), and the *Yangsheng zhi* 養生志(Record of nourishing life).[106] Thus, there can be no doubt that in the period from the Han through the Tang, there was a vibrant tradition within the Daoist religious community of concern with medicine for women, and therapies for women were significantly affected by the religion's beliefs and practices.[107]

Where does this Daoist influence manifest itself? Most obviously in dietary restrictions for pregnant women.[108] For example, the *Yang-*

---

[105] *Hanshu* 30.1778.

[106] See Catherine Despeux, "Gymnastics: The Ancient Tradition," in Livia Kohn ed., *Taoist Meditation and Longevity Techniques* (Ann Arbor: Center for Chinese Studies, University of Michigan, 1989), 225-61. For other types of Daoist medical texts, see Sakade Yoshinobu, "Daoism and the Dunhuang Regimen Texts," trans. Sumiyo Umekawa, in Lo and Cullen, eds., *Medieval Chinese Medicine*, 278-90.

[107] The first systematic study of Daoist medicine is Ge Jianmin's 蓋建民 *Daojiao yixue* 道教醫學 (Beijing: Zongjiao wenhua chubanshe, 2001), but there is no specific section in this book devoted to gynecology in the Daoist tradition. See also Xue Gongchen 薛公忱, ed., *Ru dao fo yu Zhongyi yaoxue* 儒道佛與中醫藥學 (Beijing: Zhongguo shudian, 2002).

[108] *Ishinpo*, 22.3, 873-74, "Methods for Food Prohibitions for Pregnant Women" 妊婦禁食法.

sheng yaoji states, "When a woman is pregnant she should not eat the meat of the six domestic animals, for [if she does], it will make the child not be intelligent [one text says it harms the fetus].

It also states: "Do not eat pig liver, for it will make the fetus not be born."[109]

---

[109] Other examples include the following:

It also states: Do not eat rabbit meat, for it will make [the baby] have a harelip and also the mother may not necessarily see it [the child may die].

It also states: Do not eat baby chickens or dried eel, for it will make the child have many sores.

It also states: The mother should not eat fish head, for the fetus will be damaged.

It also states: If the mother should eat hashed carp, it will make the child have many sores.

It also states: Do not eat fresh ginger, for it will make the child have extra fingers.

It also states: Do not eat dried ginger, cassia [osmanthus], or licorice, for they will make the fetus disperse and the fetus will not be at peace.

It also states: Do not drink iced broths, for it will make the fetus not be born.

It also states: Do not eat almonds and hot sweets, for they will destroy, damage, or harm the child.

It also states: Do not eat roasted sparrows with *dadou* [soybean or horsebean?] pickle, for it will make the womb leak and cause the child to have many black pimples.

It also states: Do not drink wine or eat much sparrow meat, for it will cause the child to have a licentious heart and its spirits to be disorderly.

It also states: Do not eat sparrow meat, for it will make the child have many desires [increase its desires].

It also states: Do not eat sparrow meat with sparrow brain, for it makes the child night-blind [lit., "sparrow-blind," because sparrows allegedly cannot see at night].

It also states: Do not eat sparrows with pears, for it will make the child short-tongued.

It also states: As for deer meat with plums [*Prunus mume*] and the fruit of plums [*li* 李]; if you eat them it will make the child shortsighted.

又云勿食兔肉令子脣缺亦不須見之
又云勿食雞子乾鱔魚使子多瘡
又云勿不得食魚頭胎損
又云食鯉膾令兒多瘡
又云勿食生薑令子盈指
又云勿食乾薑桂甘草令胎消胎不安
又云勿飲冰漿令胎不生
又云勿食杏仁及熱飴破損傷子
又云勿以炙雀并大豆醬食令胞漏使兒多皯皰
又云勿飲多食雀肉使子心淫精亂
又云勿食雀肉令兒多所欲
又云勿食雀肉并雀腦令人雀盲
又云勿食雀并梨子令子短舌
又云麋并梅李實食之使人清盲

The effect of this latter food also appears in the *Woming leiju chao* 倭名類聚抄 "Jibing bu" 疾病部, "Bing Lei" 病類, under *qingmang* 清盲, Ch. 7, quoting a *Shijing* 食經 (Food canon). See Morohashi Tetsuji 諸橋轍次, *Dai Kan-Wa jiten* 大漢和辭典 (Tōkyō: Taishūkan Shoten, 1976) 7.77 (6985) under *qingmang*. For a Song dynasty list of food proscriptions for pregnant women in the *yangsheng* tradition, see Zhou Shouzhong 周守忠 (fl. 1208), *Yangsheng zalei* 養生雜類, *Beijing tushuguan guji zhenben congkan*, 70.188, 9.18a-19a.

養生要集云婦人妊身不得食六畜肉令兒不聰明
又云勿食猪肝令胎不生

These dietary restrictions were clearly developed from popular beliefs and practices of late Warring States and Han times, for we find in the Mawangdui manuscript *Taichan shu* 胎產書 (Book of the generation of the fetus) similar restrictions on dietary intake according to each month of the pregnancy.[110] This manuscript is the earliest extant in a long tradition of what is known as "fetal education" (*taijiao* 胎教).[111] There is an interesting contradiction in this text: on the one hand, it states that a couple can determine the sex of a child by choosing when to copulate after the end of the menstrual flow—day one results in a boy, day two in a girl. This is because of the cosmological correlations of odd numbers with *yang* and even numbers with *yin* (in the Qin Shuihudi 睡虎地 almanac texts, even days are called "female" days and odd days "male").[112] On the other hand, the text indicates that the embryo lacked sex differentiation through the first three months of the pregnancy. As a consequence, the woman had the ability to change the sex of her child by engaging in certain activities:

> In the third month it first becomes suet, and has the appearance of a gourd. During this time it does not yet have a fixed configuration, and if exposed to things it transforms. For this reason lords, sires, and great men must not employ dwarves. Do not observe monkeys. Do not eat spring onions and ginger, and do not eat a rabbit boiled dish. [If] you wish to give birth to a boy, set out bow and arrow, … male pheasant, mount a stallion, and observe the male tiger. If you wish to give birth to a girl, wear hairpins and earrings at the waist, and wear a pearl belt. This is called "inner imaging to complete the child."[113]
> 三月始脂果隨肖效當是之時未有定儀見物而化是故君公大人毋使侏儒不觀沐猴不食蔥薑不食兔羹X欲生男置弧矢X雄雉乘牡馬觀牡虎欲生女佩簪珥紳珠子是謂內成子

[110] Harper, trans., *Early Chinese Medical Literature*, 378-80.

[111] Anne Behnke Kinney, "Dyed Silk: Han Notions of the Moral Development of Children," in Anne Behnke Kinney, ed., *Chinese Views of Childhood*, 27-28; Furth, "From Birth to Birth," 170.

[112] *Yunmeng Shuihudi Qin mu* bianxie zu 雲夢睡虎地秦墓編寫組, ed., *Yunmeng Shuihudi Qin mu* 雲夢睡虎秦墓 (Beijing: Wenwu chubanshe, 1981), plate 118, slip 759, and plates 152-53, slips 1003-04; *Yunmeng Shuihudi Qinmu* zhengli xiaozu, ed., *Shuihudi Qin mu zhujian* 睡虎地秦墓竹簡 (Beijing: Wenwu chubanshe, 2001), slip 108, 240; Liu Lexian 劉樂賢, *Shuihudi Qin jian rishu yanjiu* 睡虎地秦簡日書研究 (Taibei: Wenjin chubanshe, 1994), 355-56.

[113] Harper, trans., *Early Chinese Medical Literature*, 379, slightly modified; Ma Jixing, *Mawangdui gu yishu kaoshi* 馬王堆古醫書考釋 (Changsha: Hunan kexue jishu chubanshe, 1992), 786.

From the fourth month on, the child receives the influence of the Five Phases in succession, from Water through Earth, and in the ninth month receives the influence of stone. Ginger is avoided because it was thought to cause the child to have multiple fingers, whereas rabbit meat induced harelip, following the idea of correspondence between the external form of an object and its influence on those with whom it came into a relationship: the "resonance" (*ganying* 感應) theory popular in the Han and later times.

In fact, many of these restrictions deriving from the Daoist tradition and listed in the *Ishinpo* are also recorded by Chen Ziming in Chapter 11 of his *Furen liangfang*.[114] Yet it is this precisely this latter text that Furth holds up as paradigmatic of the new gynecology of the Song dynasty. For example, eating fresh ginger, Chen says, will result in the child having multiple fingers and being born with boils, and eating sparrow meat will result in the child being shameless and licentious.[115] Other restrictions are not recorded in earlier works, such as eating crabmeat that will result in the baby being born transversely, one of the most dangerous forms of birth, which can lead to many disasters according to Chao Yuanfang.[116] In this example, it is possible to see that the live crab's habit of crawling sideways was believed to be somehow embedded in its flesh, and this propensity would then be transferred to the baby in the womb, encouraging it, in turn, to imitate the crab's movement. Other examples represent variations on older taboos, such as those relating to soy sauce (*doujiang* 豆醬): if it is consumed with beans, it will cause the fetus to abort, and if eaten with sparrow meat, it will cause the baby's face to be covered with black freckles. Of course, the modern term for freckles, *queban* 雀斑, "sparrow spots," reflects this ancient belief.[117]

Chen also recorded a *Yunfu yaoji ge* 孕婦藥忌歌 (Song of tabooed

---

[114] Chen Ziming, *Furen liangfang jiaozhu buyi*, 336-37.

[115] Chen Ziming, *Furen liangfang jiaozhu buyi*, 337.

[116] Chao Yuanfang, *Zhubing yuanhou lun*, "Transverse Birth," 2. 1229.

[117] The famous Jin dynasty calligrapher Wang Xizhi 王羲之 (303-61) believed that such black freckles could be removed with a potion made from the excrement of the fishing cormorant (*Luci tie* 鸕鷀帖, quoted in the *Hanyu da cidian* 漢語大詞典 (Shanghai: Hanyu da cidian chubanshe, 1994), 12. 1342, under *ganzeng* 黑干黑曾), whereas the Qing scholar Wang Shixiong 王士雄 (*Suixi ju yinshi pu* 隨息居飲食譜, "Gushi lei 穀食類, Wandou 豌豆") thought that they could be removed by a compress made from peas.

medicine for pregnant women). This is a twenty-four-line poem, using the "*-ong*" rhyme at the end of each couplet and ending with the lines

> Dried ginger, garlic, chicken, and chicken eggs,
> Donkey meat and rabbit meat must not be provided.
> These are taboos that a woman absolutely must obey before giving birth:
> It is appropriate to commit this song to memory in the heart.[118]
> 乾薑蒜雞及雞子
> 驢肉兔肉不須供
> 切忌婦人產前忌
> 此歌宜記在心胸

Poems such as these occur quite frequently in the technical literature—we see them appearing, for instance, in many of the military manuals devoted to gunpowder technology—and were presumably helpful for illiterates or for those with marginal literacy to acquire access to specialized information. They could well have been the media for the transmission of a great deal of technical and esoteric knowledge over generations and centuries. As far as I am aware, these technical songs have not been the subject of any extensive research, but they certainly seem worthwhile to study for their social and technical implications, even though their aesthetic qualities may be rather less than appealing.

The other great religion that deeply influenced all levels of Chinese society and transformed its philosophical and religious beliefs, aesthetic values, social and political institutions, and religious and everyday practice between the Han and the Tang was Buddhism. It, too, had a profound influence on medicine for women. Given that the Buddhist religion, especially in its Mahāyāna form, was dedicated to the salvation of beings from the karmic cycle, it is not surprising that the Buddhists would have developed a sophisticated medical tradition. Furthermore, it is well known that the religion was very popular among women, and so it is reasonable to presume that Buddhist doctors did have treatments for women in their repertory. And perhaps much of the medical instruction was passed down orally, from nun to nun, from monk to monk, and from teacher to disciple.

Buddhists highly valued sūtras (canons) that contained the teachings of the Buddha , and so it is natural that most of the texts recovered in the hidden library at the beginning of the twentieth century

---

[118] Chen Ziming, *Furen liangfang jiaozhu buyi*, 11.337-38.

at the Dunhuang monastery complex were canonical writings. Nevertheless, quite a number of manuscripts of a medical nature were recovered in the hoard. These are to be found in the recently published, extremely valuable, volumes edited by Cong Chunyu 叢春雨 and Ma Jixing 馬繼興.[119] Used in conjunction with quotations contained in Tana's *Ishinpo*, these enable us to gain a sense of what Buddhist doctors recommended for women in experiencing childbirth.

The Dunhuang manuscript in the Stein Collection held in the London Library, S.3417, *Jiu zhuzhong sheng kunan jing* 救諸眾生苦難經 (Sūtra on saving all sentient beings from bitterness and difficulty) contains a list of ten types of death, the fifth of which is "dying in childbirth" (others are "fever," "dysentery," "eye disease," "Blood blockage," and so on).[120] Clearly, ensuring a successful, uncomplicated birth, in which the life of the mother is preserved, was of considerable importance in Buddhist medical thinking. Turning to the texts that have survived in the Dunhuang hoard, we discover that at least five are wholly or partially concerned with medicine for women, and in the chapters concerning childbirth the *Ishinpo* quotes three more, the *Zimu milu* 子母秘錄 (Secret record for mothers and children), the *Daji tuoluoni jing* 大集陀羅尼經 (Mahāsamghatadhārañī-sūtra), as well as the *Seng Shen fang* 僧深方 (Prescriptions of the monk Shen).[121]

The eminent late French sinologist Paul Demiéville noted that the Buddhist monk Zhi Yi 智顗 (538-98), the fourth patriarch of the Tiantai tradition, at the end of the sixth century, classified the etiology of diseases under six rubrics: 1) illnesses due to discord among the four elements, fire, water, air, and earth; 2) illnesses due to alimentary disturbances; 3) illnesses due to disorders in meditational exercises; 4) illnesses caused by demons that affect the body; 5) illnesses caused by Mara that affect the mind; and 6) illnesses caused by misdeeds in previous lives or the present life, among which are

---

[119] See Cong Chunyu, *Dunhuang Zhongyiyao quanshu*, and Ma Jixing, et al., eds., *Dunhuang yiyao wenxian jijiao*.

[120] *Dunhuang Zhongyiyao quanshu*, 741.

[121] A "Master Shen" (*Shen shi* 深師) is also quoted four times in the gynecology section of Wang Tao's *Waitai miyao fang*; the texts are probably the same. Gao Wenzhu, "*Waitai miyao fang* yinyong shumu wenxian kaolue" in *Waitai miyao fang*, 966-67, reckons that the women's medicine section was contained in Chapter 6 of Shen's original thirty-chapter work. For the titles of other Buddhist medical texts quoted in the *Ishinpo*, see p. 1260.

counted illnesses of the ears and genitalia as a result of gratifying sensual desires.[122] Zhi Yi argued that each of these types of illnesses was to be treated by different therapeutics. Judging by the quotations in the Dunhuang manuscripts and in the *Ishinpo*, Buddhists considered pregnant and parturient women to suffer from the first two, elemental and alimentary illnesses, and the two caused by demons, for the former are cured by prescriptions and the latter by insight exercises and incantations (*dhāraṇī*).

A close reading of the evidence reveals that the incantations were employed to prepare the birthing chamber[123] and to protect the woman at the time of birth itself and when a difficult birth was being experienced, whereas prescriptions were employed for illnesses in pregnancy and in the days following delivery. Indeed, these procedures are confirmed by the extensive quotations in the *Ishinpo* from the *Chanjing* 產經 discussed above. Even though menstrual discharge was still considered polluting as it had been in earlier times, medical writers considered that the menses could be regulated and disorders treated by the application of a standard pharmacopeia. Doctors intervened where they had previously been absent, in the actual process of delivery. But at that stage they still recognized and accepted the popular taboos and ritual procedures that had been handed down over the centuries by the women who attended the birth. Some examples of the wide range of these popular taboos and ritual procedures are presented in the following quotations. The first six derive from the *Ishinpo,* which quotes passages in order from Sun Simo and other earlier sources.[124]

> [1] *Qianjin fang* says: 'The Treatise states, "Although a parturient woman is polluted and vile (evil), yet when she is going to suffer (i.e., give birth), whether she has not yet given birth or whether she has, in both cases you should not let people from families polluted by death or mourning see her, for if you

---

[122] Mark Tatz, trans., *Buddhism and Healing: Demiéville's Article "Byō" from the Hōbōgirin* (Lanham, Md.: University Press of America, 1985), 81-82; Zhi Yi, *Mohe zhiguan* 摩訶止觀 (The great concentration), Taishō Tripitaka, *Da zangjing* 大藏經 (1911; reprint, Taibei: Xinwenfeng chuban gongsi, 1983), *ce* 64: 8A.106a-107c.

[123] For example, the *Ishinpo*, 3, 23.903, quotes the incantation from the "Birth Canon" to prepare the mat on which the woman will squat to give birth. It calls on a "King" 王 (possibly the text has omitted a graph identifying this spirit) and the Queen Mother of the West, Xiwangmu 西王母, the Red Bird of the South, Zhuque 朱雀, the Dark Warrior of the North, Xuanwu 玄武, and the Transcendents and Jade Maidens (*Xianren yunü* 仙人玉女) to protect her and keep evil ghosts and goblins away.

[124] For ease of analysis, I break up Tana's text.

do, the birth will be difficult. If she has already given birth, (and such people see her), they will harm the child.'"[125]
[2] It also states, "In general, when she is about to give birth, it is especially taboo to have many people [birth attendants] look at and watch her. Only three attendants should be at her side and wait for the birth to be completely ended and then you may tell it to others. If many others see her, everything will be difficult."[126]
[3] It also states, "When a child has come out it is taboo for all others and the mother to ask whether it is a boy or a girl. And, further, do not let the mother see or view the polluting fluids."[127]
[4] It also states, "In general, a parturient mother should take care to eat warming foods and warming medicines. One should always be aware of this, for food and drink should be like a person's flesh."[128]
[5] The *Chanjing* states, "In general, when a woman begins to give birth she should not look at herself. When she has passed (the child) over to the attendants, no one should ask whether it is a boy or a girl, and none of the attendants should say that it is a boy or a girl. For (if they do), the child will be damaged."
[6] *The Xiaopin fang* states, "In general, when a woman has given birth and is darkened (covered) with polluted blood and the fluids have not yet been cleaned up, she may not go out of doors or through the window to the location of the well or stove. It is because she shouldn't face the spirits, the god of the soil and the spirits of the ancestors."[129]

千金方云曰產婦雖是穢惡然將痛之時及未產已產并不得令死喪穢家之人來視之則生難若已 產者則傷兒子
又云凡欲產時特忌多人瞻視唯三人在旁待生悤訖了仍可告語諸人也若人衆看之無不難耳
又云兒出訖一切人及母忌問是男是女又勿令母看視穢污
又云凡產婦慎熱食熱藥常當識此飲食當如人肌
產經云凡婦人初生兒不須自視已付邊人莫問男女邊人莫言男女也兒敗
小品方云凡婦人產闇穢血露未淨不可出戶牖至井灶所也不朝神祇及祠祀也

The first passage reveals that medieval Chinese believed that those polluted by death could harm the mother and child. The second passage indicates that they believed in the possibility of danger to the child if there were more than three birth attendants. While it is

[125] This is taken from *Beiji qianjin yaofang*, 3.17b (2.242). There are a few textual variations between the passages quoted from Sun in the *Ishinpō* and the text as it is printed in the *Siku quanshu*. Tana does not quote Sun's text in its entirety.
[126] See *Beiji qianjin yaofang*, 3.18a (2.243). The current edition states "only two or three attendants."
[127] *Beiji qianjin yaofang*, 3.17b (2.242). Between this and the previous quotation, Tana omits a passage in which Sun describes how the newborn should be washed five times with fresh well water, not with warmed water.
[128] *Beiji qianjin yaofang*, 3.17b (2.242).
[129] *Ishinpo*, 3, 23.902-03, "Chanfu yongyi fa" 產婦用意法.

possible that this could be interpreted as a concern that a greater number of attendants would cause trouble by offering competing solutions to difficulties encountered during the birth, it may rather reflect ritual concerns that a gathering of more attendants might bring the attention of unwanted evil spirits who might wish to harm the newborn child. This seems to be the implication of the fifth passage quoted from the *Chanjing* which provides a "native" explanation of the reason for observing the taboo: the child will be harmed if it is spoken of right away as being a boy or a girl. Who would do the harm? The numerous powerful evil spirits, described below, that were warded off by the various ritual precautions that were taken by the mother and her family. This taboo is also recorded by Zhu Duanzhang 朱端章 (fl. 1174-89) in the Southern Song in his well-known *Weisheng jiabao chanke beiyao* 衛生家寶產科備要 (Precious family guide to protecting life in childbirth) so it was obviously a long-standing taboo that had to be observed.[130] Presumably, the naming could only be done after the child had been ritually cleansed and the appropriate amount of time (usually three days) had elapsed for the naming rite to occur. One can only speculate on the reasons why it would be considered taboo for the woman herself to look at (inspect or examine) her own polluting fluids. Perhaps it was because it was thought that she would be distressed at her own polluting and polluted state, for the last passage, from the *Xiaopin fang*, suggests that the woman might want to violate the prohibition of leaving the birthing chamber to cleanse herself with well water, but that this would result in her polluting the spirits on whom the family relied for its protection and sustenance.

One of the reviewers of this essay offers another interpretation. She/he observes that another version of the *Ishinpo* has a slightly different text at this point. This reads *Chanjing yun Fan furen chusheng er buxu zishi yi fu bianren mo wen nannü bianren mo yan nannü ye erbai* 產經云:凡婦人初生兒不須自視, 已付邊人, 莫問男女邊人, 莫言男女也, 兒敗. which the reviewer translates in part as, "the delivering mother does not need to take a look at the newborn, once it is handed to the attendants, she should not ask for its sex ..."[131] The reviewer

[130] Photographic reprint of the 1184 edition held by the Beijing University Library, *Xuxiu Siku quanshu* ed., 1007.8.

[131] See Wang Dapeng 王大鵬, Fan Youping 樊友平, et al., eds., *Ishinpo* (Shanghai: Shanghai kexue jishu chubanshe, 1998), 919.

continues, "The reason for not looking at the newborn or asking for its sex is explained by Chen Ziming in *Furen daquan liangfang*—it is to avoid the mother's emotional ups and downs in case the sex of the newborn does not meet her expectations," and argues that the passage would "be better interpreted in the context of proper midwifery than in that of pollution," as I have done. I do not have access to the original manuscript of the *Ishinpo* and therefore cannot check the exact wording. However, the Northern Song edition of Sun Simo's *Beiji qianjin yaofang*, clearly states, "When the child is completely born, everyone including the mother are all strictly tabooed from asking whether it is a boy or a girl ... Do not let the mother look at [examine] the polluting fluids" 兒生訖一切人及母皆忌問是男女 ... 勿令母看視穢污耳.[132] Sun's wording is the same in the *Siku quanshu* edition[133] and is also quoted in the *Waitai miyao fang* 外臺秘要方 (Prescriptions from the secret essentials of the Palace Library),[134] confirming the reading that I adopt. It is certainly true that Chen Ziming states (literally) that, "When the child is first born, she may not ask whether it is a girl or a boy, for fear that she will leak *qi* as a result of the talk [about the baby's sex] or her *qi* moves as a result of love or hatred, for all are capable of bringing on illness" 初產時不可問是男女, 恐因言語而泄氣, 或以愛憎而動氣, 皆能致病.[135] Yet in Chapter 16 and elsewhere in his work, Chen retains a considerable amount of the earlier lore concerning the ritual preparations of the birthing chamber and other prescriptions that draw on religious practices: for example, he provides the Buddhist incantation (*dhāraṇī*) for preparing the water to be used for purifying in the birthing process as well as the forms of the talismans to be written in red ink and stuck on the wall of the birthing chamber in cases of difficult childbirth or when the afterbirth (placenta) is not expelled.[136] This would suggest that in the case of asking whether the child is a boy or a girl, Chen is medicalizing an earlier ritual practice associated with pollution and popular religious beliefs and practices, and he omits the clause which states that identifying the sex of the child is harmful *to the child itself*. It would not do, in my opinion, to read back into

---

132 *Zhongguo yixue dacheng xuji* edition, 11.116.

133 Sun Simo, *Beiji qianjin yaofang*, 2.243; 3.18b.

134 Wang Tao, *Waitai miyao fang*, 34.676.

135 Chen Ziming, "Jiaozhu furen liangfang" 校注婦人良方, in *Zhongguo yixue dacheng* edition (Beijing: Zhongguo yiyao chubanshe, 1997), 7, 18.491.

136 Chen Ziming, "Jiaozhu furen liangfang", 7, 16.484-85.

the past Chen's recommendations and explanations in the Southern Song to interpret Tang birthing practices. Nor, might I add, do we know whether the female birth attendants and mothers in Chen's day would have accepted his interpretation of the age-old practices and beliefs at the moment of birth in the same way that he, a male Confucian literatus, did.

Doctors and medical writers recognized the necessity for the woman to create for herself a sacred ritual space in which she could give birth. This space protected her from the numerous malignant spirits in the cosmos, such as the Wandering Fetus-Killer (*riyou taisha* 日游胎殺) that came according to a strict cycle of days based on the Earthly Branches (Earth was correlated with *yin* and the Female); the spirits of the four directions, like the White Tiger; powerful astral gods; and the spirits of various days that could do her and her baby harm. In Chen Ziming's opinion in the Song, there were both Wandering Day (Sun) (*riyou taisha*) and Wandering Month (Moon) Fetus–Killer (*yueyou taisha* 月游胎殺) spirits that had to be avoided. These dangerous spirits moved around the house according to the stems of the ten-day system, on the one hand, and, on the other, the solar nodes.[137] Wang Tao, in the Tang, opined that one should set up the birthing chamber either inside the house or outside, depending on the location of these inauspicious spirits.[138]

Chao Yuanfang includes sections on birth and difficult delivery, and it is in these sections that he emphasizes the importance of following the ritual taboos and prohibitions, for failure to do so results in extremely serious consequences.

---

[137] Chen Ziming, *Furen liangfang jiaozhu*, 11.335. For example, the Wandering Month spirit was located at beds in the house at the spring equinox "Spring Begins" (*lichun* 立春), moved to the (single-leaved) doors at Excited Insects (*jingzhi* 驚蟄), to the (double-leaved) gate at Clear and Bright (*qingming* 清明), to the stove at the summer solstice (*lixia* 立夏), and so on. One had to divine for the Wandering Day spirit at the gate on *jia* 甲 and *ji* 己 days, at the mill on *yi* 乙 and *geng* 庚 days, at the well and stove on *bing* 丙 and *xin* 辛 days, in the kitchen and stable on *ding* 丁 and *ren* 壬 days, and in the granary on *wu* 戊 and *gui* 癸 days. These dangerous spirits were still believed in in late imperial times: see the entry on the Wandering Day Spirit in Chen Yongzheng 陳永正, ed., *Zhongguo fangshu da cidian* 中國方術大辭典 (Guangzhou: Zhongshan daxue chubanshe, 1991), 278, quoting Yunlu 允祿 and Zhang Zhao's 張照 *Xieji bianfang shu* 協紀辨方書 that was published by imperial order in 1743.

[138] Wang Tao, *Waitai miyao fang*, 33.665.

1. The Method of Giving Birth (*Chanfa*)

People dwell between the Three Powers [Heaven, Earth, and Man, that is, between Heaven and Earth], receive the *qi* of the Five Phases, and *yang* acts while *yin* transforms, and therefore they are caused to have children. However, although the Five Phases repeatedly produce each other, yet the hard and the soft punish and kill, and they damage and conquer each other [too]. When it comes to when [a woman] is about to give birth, then there are the days of the Wandering Day [spirits], the prohibitions and taboos of Opposing the Branches, and if [the woman] offends and goes against them, then sometimes it perversely brings on all the [various] diseases. Therefore at the time of birth she sits and rests where the birth is to take place, and she has to abide by [follow] the *qi* of the Four Seasons and Five Phases. Thus it is called the Method of Giving Birth.[139]

一 產法
人處三才之間稟五行之氣陽施陰化故令有子然五行雖復相生而剛柔刑殺互相害剋至於將產則有日遊反支禁忌若犯觸之或橫致諸病故產時坐臥產處須順四時五行之氣故謂之產法

The second prescription suggests that Chao was aware of a condition similar to the modern depression, which he considers to be caused by offending the spirits and failing to abide by the various, and frequently self-contradictory, hemerological or day prohibitions. The "methods and techniques" mentioned at the end of Chao's passage clearly were of a ritual nature that required the mother to align herself both temporally and spatially in the most auspicious setting for the dangerous, and all too often fatal, experience of giving birth:

2. Method for Guarding against Giddiness

Guarding against giddiness: In all cases, when approaching giving birth, if [a woman] has gone against and offended against all the prohibitions and taboos of the Wandering Day [Sun] [spirits] and Opposing the Branches, it will cause her Blood and *qi* not to be balanced and regulated, and it will bring about giddiness. The appearance of giddiness is that the Heart is troubled and depressed, and the *qi* is about to be terminated,[140] and so she must prepare to guard against this using methods and techniques.[141]

二 產防運法
防運者諸臨產若觸犯日遊反支諸所禁忌則令血氣不調理而致運也其運之狀心煩悶氣欲絕是也故須預以法術防之

The third passage similarly demonstrates the great concern early and medieval doctors had for speedy expulsion of the placenta and the

[139] Chao Yuanfang, *Zhubing yuanhou lun*, *juan* 43 (2.1224-25).
[140] In other words, she is about to die.
[141] Chao Yuanfang, *Zhubing yuanhou lun*, *juan* 43 (2.1225).

timely washing of the baby. But note here also Chao's suggestion that drugs should be administered immediately should the placenta not be expelled because of the obstruction of the birth canal. Here we can perhaps see male intervention at a crisis point in the delivery process and the beginning of the medicalization of practices associated with treating a retained placenta and managing its disposal. Earlier recommendations for solving the problem of a retained placenta included both ritual procedures and drugs; Chao here ignores the former and recommends the latter. But the washing in Chao's time, in my opinion, would still have been accomplished according to contemporary ritual beliefs and practices.

3. The Symptom of the Placenta not Coming out

When [a woman] gives birth and the child comes down, if the placenta does not fall, it is commonly called "resting placenta." As a result of the woman giving birth using her strength at the beginning such that she gives birth and the child comes out, yet her body is already exhausted, and she is not able use her *qi* again to give birth to the placenta, if, at the moment when she stops, external Cold affects her, then the Blood passage becomes obstructed, and so the placenta does not come out for a long time. At that point you must immediately save and cure her with prescriptions and drugs, otherwise it will be harmful to the child. The reason for this is that the placenta is linked to the baby's umbilical cord. If the placenta does not come out, then it is not possible to cut the umbilical cord and wash [the baby] at the appropriate time. If Cold *qi* harms the child, then it will become ill.

An old prescription [states] that when the placenta does not come out for a long time, there is a fear that it will injure the baby. Cut the umbilical cord according to the standard method and tie the cord with something. In addition, if there is delivery and you see that the woman who has given birth is not using thought or taking precautions and is using excessive strength, and the placenta is broken while still attached, if the placenta rises up and covers over the Heart, then it will kill the woman. If it does not cause her death, she will be ill for a long time.[142]

三 胞衣不出候
有產兒下苦胞衣不落者世謂之息胞由產婦初時用力比產兒出而體已疲頓不能更用氣產胞經停之間外冷乘之則血道否澀故胞久不出彌須急以方藥救治不爾害於兒所以爾者胞系連兒臍胞不出則不得以時斷臍浴洗冷氣傷兒則成病也
舊方胞衣久不出恐損兒者依法截臍而以物繫其帶一頭亦有產而看產人不用意慎護而挽牽甚胞系斷者其胞上掩心則斃人也縱令不死久則成病也

The Mawangdui medical texts provide the earliest evidence for the careful attention that was paid to the placenta, which was consid-

[142] Chao Yuanfang, *Zhubing yuanhou lun*, *juan* 43 (2.1225-27).

ered to have an intimate connection to the child's fate, almost a second self,[143] and a chart called *Nanfang Yu cang* 南方禹藏 (The entombment according to Yu, with south orientation) was used to determine where to bury the afterbirth to provide the baby with the best chances in life.[144] In contrast, the text from Chao above medicalizes to a certain degree the treatment of the afterbirth. The emphasis is on a retained placenta that is feared could permit the entry of disease-inducing cold vapors and could displace itself and rise up inside the woman's body, rather like the menstrual blood that was thought to rise up and transform into breast milk, and throttle her Heart, while the baby would be damaged because it was not entirely born until its accompanying afterbirth was expelled.

Medieval doctors recognized the importance for the mother to align her birth hut in the most auspicious direction for giving birth (see Appendix 1), a belief that originated before the unification of the empire.[145] They also urged the woman to ensure that her dirty blood did not pollute the ground and accepted the belief that she had to avoid giving birth to a boy or a girl in opposition to various hemerological or day systems, such as Opposing the Branch days,

---

[143] Harper, trans., *Early Chinese Medical Literature*, "Recipes for Various Cures" (*Zaliao fang* 雜療方), 367-68, translates a prescription which states that the afterbirth must be buried, after careful washing, according to strict calendro-astrological calculations, in a tightly covered pot in an unsullied *yang* location that receives long hours of sunshine.

[144] Harper, trans., *Early Chinese Medical Literature*, 374-77. For a detailed study of this text and the later history of practices associated with the afterbirth in the medical tradition, see Li Jianmin, "Mawangdui Han mu boshu 'Yu cangmai bao tu' jianzheng" 馬王堆漢墓帛書禹藏埋胞圖箋證, *Bulletin of the Institute of History and Philology* 65.4 (1994):725-832. Li includes a very useful appendix listing all the gynecology and pediatric texts that he has identified, many of which are no longer extant (pp. 792-802).

[145] In the Qin Shuihudi almanac texts, it is stated that giving birth facing north would result in the child becoming a low-caste "mean" (*jian* 賤) person, and facing northwest the child would suffer mutilating punishment. The auspicious directions of east, south, and west would result in the child being noble, wealthy, and long-lived, respectively. No doubt this was based on the notion that the north and northwest were *yin* and the other directions *yang*. See *Shuihudi Qin mu zhujian* (2001), slips 74.2, 75.2, 76.2, 236; compare *Guanju Qin Han mu jiandu*, slips 145.2, 146.2, 147.2, 148.2, 151.2, 121, and Lo Zhenyu 羅振玉, *Liusha zhuijian* 流沙墜簡 (Beijing: Zhonghua shuju, 1993), 94, where a slip from the Han dynasty suggests that facing north and west were inauspicious and would result in the child being not long-lived and poor, respectively. See also Zhang Yincheng 張寅成, *Zhongguo gudai jinji* 中國古代禁忌 (Taibei: Daoxiang chubanshe, 2000), 15-26.

which were calculated on the basis of the mother's age (see Appendix 2). They recommended the use of other magical or religious practices to ease a difficult birth, such the writing in red ink of tallies, secret forms of powerfully efficacious and exorcistic characters, and posting them on the wall of the birthing chamber, or having them burned and ingested by the expectant mother, practices that recall those of the adepts of the Celestial Masters sect of religious Daoism at the end of the Han and during the Three Kingdoms and Six Dynasties periods.[146]

Yet while they supported such ritual practices surrounding birth, doctors also advocated the use of medicinal prescriptions to ease the delivery of the child. They did not see any conflict in the two approaches. Indeed, even contemporary ordinary acupuncture therapy was carried out in accordance with hemerological prescriptions. The Chinese at that time believed that the human spirit was mobile within the body and traveled to different locations depending on the day of the month. It was therefore proscribed to needle at the point where the spirit was located on any given day (see Appendix 3).

Conclusion

In the light of the evidence presented above, I argue that the tradition of medicine for women probably began in pre-Han China, most probably on the basis of earlier practices transmitted both in written and oral form. By the middle of the Han dynasty, an extensive list of prescriptions for treating women had been compiled into a book. This text was considered important enough by scholars of the imperial court to be included in the bibliography of the imperial library. Perhaps it was read and used by the women of the imperial harem. In the early period, male doctors may have left the treatment of mothers passing through the rite of birth to female shamans, wise women, and older female members of the family. But by Sui and Tang times, male doctors were actively intervening even at

[146] Strickmann, *Magical Medicine*, Ch. 4, "Ensigillation: A Buddho-Taoist Technique of Exorcism," 167-68, translates a Dunhuang text which provides details of an extremely efficacious seal of Guanyin (Avalokiteśvara), which was to be ingested by women desiring children on the Buddha's birthday, the eighth day of the fourth month, a remedy that ensured the production of a girl or a boy, whichever the mother desired.

this crucial and ritually important stage, despite the pollution generated by the woman's birth fluids. Possibly, she was considered polluting by her change of status from childless woman to mother and thus to full participant in the ritual and social life of her husband's family and lineage.[147]

The trajectory of women's medicine indicates that it was deeply influenced by a variety of philosophical, religious, and popular practices, from magic and popular religious ideas in ghosts and powerful gods and spirits, to Five Phase and *yin/yang* thinking, to the doctrine of systematic correspondence and resonance, to the beliefs and practices of the Daoist and Buddhist religions. It is incumbent upon us to try to interpret the cultural meanings of these beliefs and practices, and in this paper I have tried to make a start on this project. Much work still remains to be done, and many questions remain unanswered.

But we can conclude that, over the centuries, doctors became confident enough to prescribe a wide range of herbal drugs in a wide range of combinations, to be administered to the patient in a range of forms. Their pharmacopeia constantly grew, even as they attempted to treat an increasingly large number of medical problems and even as they developed more complex theoretical systems to explain the diseases they encountered and to organize their therapies. They rarely applied acupuncture to treat problems of expectant, parturient, and postpartum women. Finally, medicine in China began to be gendered at least as early as the Sui and Tang dynasties. It was therefore on the basis of a very rich and complex tradition that Song and later doctors built their own edifice of gynecology, a tradition that remains alive and well to this day.

---

[147] Li Zhende, "Han Tang zhijian qiuzi yifang shitan."

Appendix 1

Ishinpo, "Chanfu anchan lu fa" 產婦安產廬法 (Method for a pregnant woman to set up her birth hut), 23.903, reads:

> The *Chanjing* states: The directions according to the month for a peaceful birth hut that are auspicious [are as follows]:

Month	Auspicious Direction
1, 6, 7, 11	Facing southeast
2, 3, 4, 5, 8, 9, 10, 12	Facing southwest

> In general, when constructing a birth hut, do not use buckthorn or jujube, or barbed or curved poles. Furthermore, it is prohibited to dwell or give birth beneath sheaves of wheat or beneath a water tree (*shuishu* 水樹) [a tree that I have not been able to identify, although it might be a willow]. That is very inauspicious. Also, do not approach the stove or the sacrifices: that is also very inauspicious.

> 產經云按月之方安產廬吉正月六月七月十一月作廬一戶皆東南向吉
> 二月三月四月五月八月九月十月十二月作廬一戶皆西南向吉
> 凡作產廬無以棗棘子鋌戟杖又禁居生麥稼水樹下大凶又勿近灶祭亦大凶

Here the prescriptions seem to prohibit using wood taken from plants that have something sharp about them, presumably because of the belief that the sharpness, and thus pain and difficulty, will be transferred to the woman as she gives birth. Also evident in the prohibition at the end is the belief that a parturient woman would pollute the stove, where all the household food was prepared, and would harm the stove-god who looked after the family and reported its actions to the Lord-on-High at the end of the year, and would incur the wrath of the gods and ancestors, if she appeared at a sacrifice. So the confinement of a parturient mother in the birth chamber was not just for her own health and safety, but for the protection of the whole family and for the gods and ancestors that the family worshipped.

Appendix 2

Ishinpo, "Chanfu fanzhi yueji fa" 產婦反支月忌法 (The method for a birthing woman with respect to "opposing the branches" and the monthly taboos), 23.901-02, provides details on this *fanzhi* method as it related to birthing. The term *fanzhi* appears in the *Hou Hanshu* "Biography of Wang Fu," 49.1640). This is an excerpt from Wang Fu's 王符 *Qianfu Lun* 潛夫論 "Airi" 愛日 *pian* 18, which states that Emperor Mingdi 明帝(r. 58-75)objected to the practice of the people not submitting memorials on *fanzhi* days. This also appears in the *Zizhi tongjian* 資治通鑒 "Han Ji," 漢紀 under Mingdi, eighteenth year of Yongping 永平 (75 CE, the last year of Mingdi's life) (Beijing: Zhonghua shuju, 1992), *juan* 45, 2.1465-66, where the quotation is the same as Wang Fu's *Qianfu lun*, and the commentary states the same as the commentary in the *Hou Hanshu*. Both indicate that the "Yin Yang shu" (Treatise on *yin yang*) is the source of the explanation of the *fanzhi* day system. See *Qianfu lun jian* 潛夫論箋, commentary by Wang Jipei 汪繼培, subcommentary by Peng Duo 彭鐸 (Beijing: Zhonghua shuju, 1979), 4.221. The commentary explains that the system uses the day reckoning according to the twelve earthly branches (*dizhi* 地支): "You use the first day of the month as the regulator. When *xu* 戌 (b11) and *hai* 亥 (b12) are the first day of the month, day one is *fanzhi*; when *shen* 申 (b9) and *you* 酉 (b10) are the first day of the month, day two is *fanzhi*; when *wu* 午 (b7) and *wei* 未 (b8) are the first day of the month, day 3 is *fanzhi*; when *chen* 辰 (b5) and *si* 巳 (b6) are the first day of the month, day 4 is *fanzhi*; when *yin* 寅 (b3) and *mao* 卯 (b4) are the first day of the month, day 5 is *fanzhi*; when *zi* 子 (b1) and *chou* 丑 (b2) are the first day of the month, day 6 is *fanzhi*. See *Yin Yang shu*)." Obviously Mingdi was not successful, for Yan Zhitui 顔之推 (531-91) also noted the taboos of the *fanzhi* system when he wrote in his *Yanshi jiaxun* 顔氏家訓, *juan* 7, *pian* 19, "Za Yi" 雜藝, "When it reaches the *fanzhi* day, do not travel to the borders as you will encounter harm." See Wang Liqi 王利器 ed., *Yanshi jiaxun jijie* 顔氏家訓集解 (Taibei: Mingwen shuju, 1990), 521. Teng Ssu-yü, *Family Instructions for the Yen Clan: Yen-shih Chia-hsün* (Leiden: Brill, 1968), 204, translates *fanzhi* as "reversing the combination of Stems (*kan* [干]) and Branches (*chih* [支])."

The *Ishinpo* quotes the *Chanjing* in saying that if a parturient woman or a woman giving suck disobeys the *fanzhi*, it is extremely dangerous (literally, "ten deaths"), and she absolutely must take precautions. If she happens to violate the branches in a month, she has to stand on ox hide (cowhide) or on ashes and not let polluted water or blood or vile things touch the earth. If they touch the earth, then people will be killed. Furthermore, when washing and purifying herself she has always to use vessels to hold the fluids. That is, she presumably must not wash in pools or streams. This would be to prevent the pollution from soiling the earth.

Then the text lists the *fanzhi* on the basis of the years, the age of the woman, when giving birth to a girl, and the *fanzhi* days: this is the same as in the *Qianfu lun* and *Hou Hanshu*.

She must not give birth in violation of the following rules: that is, in a *zi* year, she must not give birth on a *shen* day in the seventh month.

Year	month	location of *fanzhi*
zi 子	7	*shen* 申
chou 丑	8	*you* 酉
yin 寅	9	*xu* 戌
mao 卯	10	*hai* 亥
chen 辰	11	*zi* 子
si 巳	12	*chou* 丑
wu 午	1	*yin* 寅
wei 未	2	*mao* 卯
shen 申	3	*chen* 辰
you 酉	4	*si* 巳
xu 戌	5	*wu* 午
hai 亥	6	*wei* 未

Age of mother	month	location of *fanzhi*
13	7	*shen* 申
14	8	*you* 酉
15	9	*xu* 戌
16	10	*hai* 亥
17	11	*zi* 子
18	12	*chou* 丑
19	1	*yin* 寅
20	2	*mao* 卯
21	3	*chen* 辰
22	4	*si* 巳
23	5	*wu* 午
24	6	*wei* 未
25	7	*shen* 申
26	8	*you* 酉
27	9	*xu* 戌
28	10	*hai* 亥

Age of mother	month	location of *fanzhi*
29	11	*zi* 子
30	12	*chou* 丑
31	1	*yin* 寅
32	2	*mao* 卯
33	3	*chen* 辰
34	4	*si* 巳
35	5	*wu* 午
36	6	*wei* 未
37	7	*shen* 申
38	8	*you* 酉
39	9	*xu* 戌
40	10	*hai* 亥
41	11	*zi* 子
42	12	*chou* 丑
43	1	*yin* 寅
44	2	*mao* 卯
45	3	*chen* 辰
46	4	*si* 巳
47	5	*wu* 午
48	6	*wei* 未
49	7	*shen* 申

The *fanzhi* when giving birth to a girl according to the *Ishinpō*:

Year	month of *fanzhi*
zi 子	1
hai 亥	2
xu 戌	3
you 酉	4
shen 申	5 (6)
wu 午	6
wei (*wu*) 未	7
si 巳	8
chen 辰	9
mao 卯	10
yin 寅	11
chou 丑	12

The *Wutai miyao*, *juan* 33, 663-65, quotes an even more complicated version of the *fanzhi* system developed by the noted Tang doctor Cui Zhiti. In this system, the age of the mother from thirteen through forty-nine—though it is doubtful that a woman of that age would be able to give birth—is correlated with an even broader number of factors. They are, first, the year in which her fortune is to change (*xingnian* 行年) calculated according to the years reckoned by the stems and branches from number 57 *gengshen* 庚申 for a thirteen-year-old mother backwards to *jiashen* 甲申 for a forty-nine-year-old mother. This is followed by the *fanzhi* always reckoned by two months. In these two months she should not allow her blood to pollute the earth, for that will cause the child to die in her belly or the birth to be difficult. She must first scatter the earth with ashes and grass and then cover it over with a mat made of horse, donkey, or ox hide. She can give birth on top of that, and it will be auspicious. Then "Misfortune and Harm" (*huohai* 禍害) and "Cutting off Fate or Life" (*jueming* 絕命) are calculated by direction and trigram from the *Yijing* 易經 (Book of changes). The prospective mother must not urinate, defecate, or give birth facing these directions, otherwise it is inauspicious, and the blood will not stop after delivery. Here one can see that giving birth is considered equivalent to evacuating, and all three are believed to be polluting.

Next comes "Live *Qi*" (*sheng qi* 生氣), also reckoned according to direction and trigram, which is the direction that she should face when giving birth to ensure long life for the baby and auspiciousness for both mother and child. The next correlation uses directions and the Five Phases. The mother should summon a master (*shi* 師), whose gender is not specified, from a particular direction wearing clothing of a correlated color, that she should match in her own clothing, to oversee the birth. This is followed by the direction she should lay her head when resting. Next comes "Suspending the corpse" (*xuanshi* 懸尸), reckoned by days enumerated according to their stem-and-branch coordinates. On the specified days it is considered inauspicious to hang up ropes. The text also states that is auspicious to hang up ropes made from horse reins. Since mothers would normally give birth in a vertical position, I suspect that these ropes would be suspended from the ceiling and would be held by the mother when she was giving birth. If this is so, it is noteworthy that it would imply that the mother is referred to as a "corpse."

Finally, there are the "Closing the Belly" (*bidu* 閉肚) and the "Eight Strong Men" (*bazhuang* 八壯), which Cheng Jingtong 程敬通 (1597-?) thinks is probably a copyist's mistake for "Entering the Belly" (*rudu* 入肚), since one edition reads the latter graphs (p. 665, note 3). Both of these are reckoned according to the directions as indicated by the positions of the ten stems. On days of "Closing the Belly" when the mother is approaching delivery or has given birth and is "doing the month" of seclusion, she should not face that direction to urinate, defecate, or throw away dirty water. If she does, it will either cause her birth tract to close up and the birth will be difficult, or she will lose her color, her belly will ache, her face will become paralyzed and yellow (jaundiced?), her navel will become twisted and painful, and it will be difficult to swallow, all of which are reckoned to be inauspicious. The mother must not open the screen or gate to her birth hut or give birth towards the directions indicated under the rubric "Eight Strong Men" or "Entering the Belly," for that is extremely inauspicious and would result in the birth tract closing up and a difficult birth.

Appendix 3

The *Renshen riji* 人神日忌 (Taboo days for the human spirit) survived in the Dunhuang library and is now preserved in the Bibliothèque Nationale, Paris, as Pelliot 3247 (P.3247) (Cong Chunyu, ed., *Dunhuang Zhongyiyao quanshu* 敦煌中醫藥全書, 220). This manuscript, written on both sides of the roll below the *Sifen lüjie mo* 四分律羯磨 on the recto side and the *Da Tang Tongguang si nian juli* 大唐同光四年具曆 (Complete calendar for the fourth year of Tongguang [926] of the Great Tang Dynasty) on the verso, is similar to one that appears in the *Xinji beiji jiujing* 新集備急灸經 and specifies the location in the human body of the human spirit on different days of the month. It was taboo to apply acupuncture at the spot where the spirit was located on a particular day.

Day	Location of the Human Spirit
1	Big toe
2	Outer side of the ankle
3	Inner thigh
4	Waist
5	Mouth
6	Little finger
7	Inner side of the ankle
8	Front of the ankle (?)
9	Tip of the spine
10	Back of the waist
11	Bridge (?) of the nose
12	Hairline
13	Teeth
14	Stomach tube
15	Entire body
16	Chest
17	Throat (?) *Qi chong* 氣沖
18	Inner thigh
19	Foot
20	Inner side of the ankle
21	Little finger
22	Outer side of the ankle
23	Liver
24	*Yangming* 陽明 point on the hand
25	*Yangming* point on the foot
26	Chest
27	Knee
28	Genitals
29	Knee cap (?)
30	Sole of the foot

"TEN TIMES MORE DIFFICULT TO TREAT" FEMALE BODIES IN MEDICAL TEXTS FROM EARLY IMPERIAL CHINA[1]

BY

SABINE WILMS
(Paradigm Publications)

Abstract

This paper examines the interpretation of female bodies by male medical authors in post-Han China, investigating medical theories and practices as reflected in the applied medical literature of "prescriptions for women." Between the Han and Song periods, this paper argues, the negative association of the female body with the vague category of pathologies "below the girdle," referring most notably to conditions of vaginal discharge, was replaced with a more positive focus on menstruation, which symbolized regular and predictable cycles of generativity and free flow. As male physicians came to recognize the female body as gendered and accepted the need for a specialized treatment of women, menstruation became the window through which they gained access to the hidden processes inside the female body. By "balancing/regulating the menses," they learned to treat and prevent such dreaded chronic conditions as infertility, susceptibility to cold, or general emaciation and weakness, all which were seen as related to the female reproductive processes. Thus, the practice of menstrual regulation ultimately served to ensure female fertility and the continuation of the family line.

Introduction

This article contributes to the study of women and gender in post-Han China by focusing on the female body as it was treated and interpreted in medical texts between the Han and Song periods (third to

[1] This article is based on my paper, "From Leaking Discharge to Irregular Menstruation: The Conceptualization of Female Pathology in Medieval China," presented at the Association for Asian Studies Annual Meeting, March 4-7, 2004, San Diego, as part of the panel, 'Constructing Paradigms of Female Pathology in Medieval and Late Imperial China.' I would like to thank the other participants of the panel, Charlotte Furth, Bridie Andrews, Vijaya Deshpande, and Yi-Li Wu, as well as several listeners from the audience, for critical comments and suggestions for further research.

Also available online – www.brill.nl

tenth centuries CE). In other words, it investigates the way in which male authors of technical medical literature dealt with the physicality of the female body and the fundamental problem of its otherness in the context of medical diagnosis and treatment.

As long as women have given birth, the female body has served as an obvious yet multidimensional source of a culture's metaphors for cosmology, creation, gender and family relations, and even politics. At the same time, medical, moral, religious, and other discourses on the female body have used it as a vehicle for expressing larger cultural values and agendas, whether consciously or not.[2] The direct and reciprocal relationship between conceptions of the female body and gender roles hardly needs to be stressed. Naturally, ideas about the female body are, in any culture or context, closely connected to a society's view of childbirth, since the most obvious difference between the sexes is that women give birth and men don't. But, as Thomas Laqueur pointed out in his study of reproductive biology in seventeenth-century England, "the cultural construction of the female in relation to the male, while expressed in terms of the body's concrete realities, was more deeply grounded in assumptions about the nature of politics and society."[3]

Medical discourse, in early imperial China as elsewhere, is unique in that it presumes to address the body's "concrete realities" for the sole purpose of alleviating its suffering, rather than as an indirect metaphor for cosmological, political, moral, or other themes. Thereby, it provides a window into a culture's values and ideas on the deepest level of embodiment. Recognizing the potential of the female body as both a source and a site for the expression of ideology, this article therefore approaches post-Han Chinese medical texts with the following questions: What functions of the female body did the authors consider as natural, as ideal, or as pathological, and as weakening or as strengthening for the general constitution of women? What conditions did they recognize as specifically female pa-

[2] One only needs to look at recent political debates on abortion in the United States. See also Emily Martin, *The Woman in the Body: A Cultural Analysis of Reproduction* (Boston: Beacon Press, 1987), an analysis of the rich metaphors underlying modern biomedical descriptions of reproductive processes in the female body and their relationship to dominant social, political, and economic values.

[3] Thomas Laqueur, "Orgasm, Generation, and the Politics of Reproductive Biology," *Representations* 14 (1986):1-41, 16.

thologies in need of gender-specific treatments? Or, more broadly, what aspects of the female body were regarded as specifically female and therefore as instrumental in defining and justifying male physicians' specialized approach to women's bodies? Last but not least, the question which has occupied innumerable healers and thinkers in all ages and cultures since the alleged creation of Eve out of Adam's rib: How is the female body related to the male, and implied in this, how is woman related to man?

To answer these questions, the core of this article traces the stages by which the male authors[4] of a technical literature of *furen fang* 婦人方 (prescriptions for women)[5] gradually came to conceptualize the female body as separate from the male in post-Han China. For this purpose, I will first review the medical model of androgyny by which male and female bodies were related to each other in the early Han medical classics. This androgynous view of the human body was elaborated most succinctly in theoretical medical classics like the *Huangdi neijing* 黃帝內經 (Inner classic of the Yellow Emperor). The tight correlations and parallel functioning of human, cosmic, and political bodies in the theory of systematic correspondences from the Han dynasty on offered, in the abstractions of *yin* and *yang*, an evocative metaphor from which to interpret the difference between the sexes. Challenging the gender-neutral view of the human body in the early classics, already in the seventh century, Sun Simiao (孫思邈 581?-682) wrote in a famous collection of prescriptions that "women's disorders are ten times more difficult

---

[4] I consciously avoid calling most authors of early Chinese medical texts "physicians." While it is clear that these members of the literate elite were personally engaged in the maintenance and improvement of their own and their family's health, their active and professional involvement in clinical practice is often subject to debate. The composition of medical literature could therefore in many cases have been limited to the collection, compilation, and synthesis of previous texts, becoming an endeavor more reflective of the author's literary skills and access to libraries and texts than of his medical knowledge.

[5] This is the standard term by which treatments that address conditions of the adult female body are referred to in the medical literature. The literal translation from the Chinese would be "prescriptions for wives," but the content makes it clear that this category also includes nuns, widows, and other unmarried women. Thus, it refers to women from the time of menarche on. Throughout this article, I translate *fang* as "prescriptions," but it should be noted that this term includes not only medicinal formulas and acupuncture instructions, but also common household recipes, religious instructions, and physical manipulations like massage and childbirth positions.

to treat than men's."[6] In the two main sections of this article, I will compare and contrast the early Han theoretical model of androgyny with a clinically applied discourse on what the authors saw as the lived experience of the female body as it emerged over the following centuries in a technical literature of "prescriptions for women." First, I will analyze the development of female pathology, as it is reflected in the categorizations and etiological interpretations of women's conditions. Second, I will look more closely at the origin of ideas about female Blood[7] and menstruation.

During the Song dynasty, the recognition that women required therapeutic strategies that were categorically different from men's resulted in the formation of a true gynecology or *fuke* 婦科. For the purposes of this article, I employ the term "gynecology" in the sense of a professionalized medical field that specializes in the treatment of women and exists separate from and in addition to obstetrics, or *chanke* 產科. In China, the key factor in this process was the realization of the central role of *xue* 血 (Blood) and, directly related to this, menstruation, in the female body, which replaced earlier notions of women as defined by conditions of *daixia* 帶下 (below the girdle). This innovative approach allowed for a holistic and theoretically grounded conception of the female body. It also stimulated the development of the sophisticated diagnoses, complex treatments, and preventative measures, which traditional Chinese gynecologists employ to this day.

Androgyny in the Chinese Medical Classics

Any depiction of a concept as culturally inscribed, metaphorically rich, polyvalent, and yet personal as the female body is fraught with difficulties. These are only compounded by problems of translation into another language, culture, and time. At first sight, the Han-period Chinese medical classics appear to express what Lisa Raphals in her study of women in early Chinese medical literature consid-

[6] Sun Simiao, *Beiji qianjin yaofang* 備急千金要方, 250 *juan* (ca. 652; reprint, Beijing: Huaxia chubanshe, 1996), 2.1.

[7] I capitalize the term when it refers not to the biomedical concept of blood but to the Chinese concept of *xue* 血. This includes not only our notion of blood, but also such substances as the nourishment to the fetus in the womb, breast milk, and abdominal masses.

ers a "fairly consistent rejection of sexual difference in medical diagnosis and treatment, based on *yin-yang* theories."[8] Speaking for a later period and in the context of a specialized gynecological literature, Charlotte Furth, in her analysis of gender in traditional Chinese medicine between the Song and Ming periods, introduces the notion of androgyny.[9] Well aware of the complexity of Chinese ideas about culturally constructed gender and biologically based sex, she begins her study by creating a normative and ahistorical "Yellow Emperor's Body" on the basis of the Han to Tang medical classics: "Unlike the Galenic human 'one sex' patterned on a male norm, the Yellow Emperor's Body is more truly androgynous, balancing *yin* and *yang* functions in everyone." [10] It reflects an androgynous ideal of generative power with homologous functions of *yang* essence and *yin* Blood in both sexes. In this characterization, Furth successfully emphasizes the fluidity of Chinese conceptions of the body which, in late imperial times, lead, for example, to discussions on male uteruses and lactating scholars.[11]

Furth's application of the concept of androgyny to describe the relationship between female and male bodies in the medical classics suggests a view which differs sharply from the one discussed in the main part of this paper below, which is based on the applied literature of "prescriptions for women." The following paragraphs will therefore look more closely at the origins of this earlier paradigm of androgyny, which undoubtedly also informed the approach of the authors of the early gynecological texts treated below.

On the most general level, it is common knowledge that Chinese culture has long associated women's physical bodies, as well as such gendered personality traits as softness, receptiveness, weakness, hierarchical inferiority, and yielding, with *yin*, while masculine bodies and attributes have been associated with *yang*. In the system of

---

[8] Lisa Raphals, *Sharing the Light: Representations of Women and Virtue in Early China* (Albany: State University of New York Press, 1998), 192-93.

[9] Charlotte Furth, *A Flourishing Yin: Gender in China's Medical History, 960-1665* (Berkeley: University of California Press, 1999).

[10] Furth, *A Flourishing Yin*, 46.

[11] Furth, *A Flourishing Yin*, Ch. 6, " 'Nourishing Life': Ming Bodies of Generation and Longevity," 187-223; and Yi-Li Wu, "A Vessel of Blood, A Gate of Life: Metaphors of Uterine Function and the Construction of Female Illness in Ming-Qing Gynecology" (Paper Presented at the Association for Asian Studies Annual Meeting, March 4-7, 2004, San Diego.

correlative thinking, which originated in the third century BCE and became pervasive in all aspects of Chinese culture during the Han dynasty, *yin* and *yang* symbolized a basic duality that linked the macrocosm to all kinds of microcosms, from the universe to the body politic to the human body, in systematic, perceivable, and predictable cycles of change.[12] Parallel to the macrocosm, any microcosm was seen as oscillating between these two dynamic polarities in a continual and dynamic relationship, rather than as resting in absolute binary categories. As the *Daodejing* states, "Everything embodies *yin* and embraces *yang*. Through blending these vital energies, they attain harmony."[13] In the practical application of this system of natural philosophy, it was the role of educated men, whether physicians, emperors, philosophers, or astrologers, to maintain or restore a state of balance and harmony between the poles of *yin* and *yang* within a microcosm and in relation to the macrocosm.

Also—and this is significant for our understanding of early Chinese medical texts—any discourse on one of the correlated microcosms functioned simultaneously as a statement of cosmological and political significance. Natural philosophers, scientists and other technical specialists were sought-after visitors at the feudal and then imperial courts of the Warring States and Han periods because of their insights into a particular microcosm and therefore, by logical extension, into the larger picture.[14] Continuing into the Tang dynasty, the political involvement of such medical authors as Sun Simiao provides ample proof that they were well aware of the cosmological and political implications of their theories. Thus, they studied and constructed medical discourse as just one of many avenues

---

[12] For a historically informed description of the system of correlative thinking as applied to early Chinese medicine, see Paul U. Unschuld, *Medicine in China: A History of Ideas*, Ch. 3, "Unification of the Empire, Confucianism, and the Medicine of Systematic Correspondence" (Berkeley: University of California Press, 1985), 51-100. For a discussion of *yin* and *yang* in the context of gender in Chinese medicine, see Furth, *A Flourishing Yin*, Ch. 1, "The Yellow Emperor's Body," 19-58, and Raphals, *Sharing the Light*, Chs. 6, "Yin and Yang" and 7, "Yin-Yang in Medical Texts," 139-94.

[13] *Daodejing* 42. Translated in Robin R. Wang, ed., *Images of Women in Chinese Thought and Culture* (Indianapolis: Hackett Publishing Co., 2003), 69.

[14] For a comparison between Chinese and Greek patterns of patronage and their influence on scientific inquiry, see Geoffrey Lloyd and Nathan Sivin, *The Way and the Word: Science and Medicine in Early China and Greece* (New Haven: Yale University Press, 2002), esp. "Macrocosm and Microcosm," 214-26.

for the grand enterprise of "nurturing life" and based their medical practice on inspiration from intuitive insights into the macrocosm at large.

Given these added dimensions of medical texts, the interpretation of the female body and its relationship to the male body is fraught with multiple meanings. To summarize the standard view of Chinese medical theory in the early classics, physical sex is only one factor to affect the balance of *yin* and *yang* in any body. The dominance of *yin* in a female body and of *yang* in a male body is counteracted or reinforced by age (*yang* being young and *yin* being old), climate and weather (*yin* being winter/cold/wet and *yang* being summer/hot/dry), or diet, to name just a few examples. And to complicate matters further, *yin* and *yang* coexist within each body in sometimes complementary, sometimes hierarchical or encompassing pairs: For example, the locations of inside/outside and below/above; the vital fluids Blood and *qi*, which are further differentiated into the relationship between essence and *qi* and Blood and essence; the six *yin* and six *yang* channels; and the six viscera and bowels are each associated with *yin* and *yang*, respectively. In any human body, the kidneys, associated with water among the five phases, and with generative vitality and primordial *qi*, are the most *yin* of the internal organs. They are closely linked to the genitals, often referred to, in both men and women, as *yin chu* 陰處 (*yin* place) or *yin qi* 陰器 (*yin* instruments). Both male and female bodies are marked by equivalent generative functions that are associated with the kidneys and the genitals.

The Han period medical classics like the *Huangdi neijing* and the *Nanjing* 難經 (Classic of difficult issues) already express this view of the human body, treating *yin* and *yang* primarily not as references to sexual differences, but as basic polarities to describe the correlations of any human body to the macrocosm. Regarding any difference between the sexes, the most significant reference in the *Huangdi neijing* is the account of the life cycles of male and female bodies: They differ only in the fact that women, being associated with *yin* and therefore with odd numbers, mature in multiples of seven, and men, being associated with *yang* and even numbers, mature in cycles of eight. Otherwise, men and women develop homologous bodies with equivalent functions, characterized by the rise and decline of their reproductive capacities rather than by gendered anatomical features like beards or breasts.[15] Another notion mentioned sporadically in the classics is the fact that female and male bodies manifest different pulses, such as, in the *Huangdi neijing*, on opposite sides of the body since *yin* is associated with right and *yang* with left,[16] or, in the *Nanjing*, being stronger in different locations on the wrist.[17] Other than in these isolated instances, however, the human body discussed in the early theoretical literature is for the most part a sexually neutral one and can therefore truly be called "androgynous."

Thus the Han-period classics present us with a medical paradigm in which female bodies are related to male bodies in a homologous relationship. Both sexes are seen as equally valid variations along a continuum, the ideal of which is not situated at either the male or the female pole, but at the center. As an ideal, the early classics thus construct an androgynous body which transcends sexual differentiation and embodies, in both sexes, the generative power that results from a perfect state of harmony between *yin* and *yang*. In addition, the axis of masculinity or femininity is only one of many to affect this balance and is counteracted or reinforced by others such as age, diet, lifestyle, seasons, location, and so forth. This ideal human body, which, in both sexes, contains male and female functions of generation and gestation, then becomes a powerful metaphor to describe the cosmic process of creation. Based on a linkage between human birth and cosmogenesis, the reproductive capacities of female bodies are idealized in the early philosophical, cosmological, and medical literature and extended metaphorically from female bodies not only to male bodies, but to cosmic, political, and other bodies as well.

Nonetheless, regardless of the philosophical foundations, author's background, and intended audience of a certain medical text, medicine is always more than a theoretical exploration of macrocosmic processes at the site of the human body. As it was defined in the earliest Chinese dictionary in the second century CE, "*yi: zhi bing gong ye* 醫: 治病工也 (medicine is the skill of treating disease)."[18] And

---

[15] For a translation and interpretation, see Furth, *A Flourishing Yin*, 45-48.

[16] *Suwen* 素問 15.2, translated in Raphals, *Sharing the Light*, 188.

[17] *Nanjing*, "The Nineteenth Difficult Issue," trans. and annotated in Paul U. Unschuld, *Medicine in China: Nan-ching, the Classic of Difficult Issues* (Berkeley: University of California Press, 1986), 259-67.

[18] Xu Shen 許慎, *Shuowen jiezi* 說文解字 (early second century CE; reprint, Henan: Zhongyuan nongmin chubanshe, 2000), 14.1401.

when early Chinese doctors were confronted with the task of treating female bodies, the clinical realities of a body that was so obviously affected by the specifically female processes of reproduction and gestation forced them to look beyond the androgynous ideal. The realization that women did in fact suffer from conditions which were categorically different from men's thus led to the birth of gynecology. As would be expected, the technical literature of prescription collections, originating from and aimed at a concrete application in clinical practice, reflected this awareness more clearly than the theoretical treatises in which the macrocosmic significance of bodily processes was discussed.

Female Pathology as a Basis for Gender Difference

In the following pages, I will introduce the reader to a very different perspective, based on sources concerned not with theoretical statements about the female body as a metaphor of cosmic creation or symbol of the balance between *yin* and *yang*, but with the embodied experience of women's suffering in medical practice. The female body described here is characterized by uncontrollable and often life-endangering leaking and flooding of vital fluids from orifices above and below, by erratic emotions and disabling dreams which fluctuate periodically, and by its openness and vulnerability to such pathogenic substances as wind, cold, and postpartum blood, in addition to chronic vacuity and weakness that result from the ravages of pregnancy, childbirth, and lactation.

The earliest reference to medical treatment of women is found in the second-century BCE *Shiji* biography of the mythological itinerant physician Bian Que 扁鵲. In this text, the term *daixia yi* 帶下醫 (physician treating conditions below the girdle) is used to refer to a person engaged in the medical treatment of women, indicating that the association of *daixia* with the female body must go back at least to the second century BCE.[19] The term *daixia* becomes a key

[19] Bian Que's biography is found in Ch. 105 of the *Shiji* 史記, which is titled *Bian Que Canggong liezhuan* 扁鵲倉公列傳 (Biographies of Bian Que and Canggong). For an explanation of the term *daixia yi* here, see Wang Shaozeng 王紹增 and Zhang Tianzhu 張天柱, eds., *Yi guwen baipian shiyi* 醫古文百篇釋譯 (Harbin: Heilongjiang kexue jishu chubanshe, 1995), 95, n. 99. The editors paraphrase it as *fuke yisheng* 婦科醫生 (physician of gynecology), explaining that "the conditions which trouble

notion in the development of gynecology over the subsequent centuries when it is used increasingly in the more restrictive technical sense of "vaginal discharge." The following paragraphs will describe this development in detail through a close reading, in chronological order, of the three earliest major primary sources on women's medical treatment.

Daixia (Below the girdle): *The Jingui yaolüe*

The first text to accord a separate section to women's conditions is the Eastern Han formulary *Jingui yaolüe* 金匱要略 (Essentials of the golden casket) by Zhang Ji 張機.[20] The three short chapters on women, constituting about ten percent of the whole text, are located at the very end of the book, followed only by chapters on miscellaneous disorders and dietary taboos. After two chapters on pregnancy and postpartum conditions, the third chapter covers miscellaneous gynecological conditions, apparently tagged on and compiled with no particular organizational scheme. As Zhang himself points out in the middle of this section, women's disorders located in the upper and middle sections of the body—like vomiting, lung abscesses, flank pain, binding heat, or scaly skin—are no different from men's and are therefore to be treated with prescriptions found in the general sections of his text. It is only conditions "below the girdle," *daixia*, specifically those related to the reproductive and digestive systems, which require special gender-specific treatment. The following statement is an isolated and rudimentary trace of etiological ideas which came to be elaborated and differentiated in great detail in later gynecological texts:

> Women's disorders are caused by vacuity, accumulated cold, and bound *qi*. This constitutes the various [conditions of] interrupted menstruation. If it becomes chronic, cold and Blood gather together and bind with each other, the entrance to the uterus [is affected by] cold damage and the [flow of *qi* in the] channels and network vessels congeals and solidifies.[21]

---

women (menstruation, discharge, pregnancy, and childbirth) are mostly related to the region below the *daimai* 帶脈 (girdle channel)." However, since the early medical literature does not yet emphasize the role of this channel in women-related etiologies, the term refers rather to the location of a woman's girdle itself.

[20] Zhang Ji, *Jingui yaolüe* (Eastern Han; reprint, Shanghai: Shanghai kexue jishu chubanshe, 1991).

[21] Zhang, *Jingui yaolüe*, 22.667.

In addition to this etiology of blocked flow and pain due to vacuity cold, however, Zhang cites with equal frequency an etiology of "heat entering the Blood chamber," most often due to contracting wind evil. Similar to his literal use of the term *daixia* as the region "below the girdle," *xueshi* 血室 (Blood chamber) is here simply a general term referring to the location where female Blood is created, stored, and distributed. The external pathogens of wind and cold, which continue to play a central role in Chinese gynecology to this day, are already known to cause an irregular menstrual flow as well as mental instability which, Zhang stresses, is a problem related to *daixia*, here in the sense of "women's disorders," not one caused by spirits. It is also important to note that Zhang never mentions the pathologies of abdominal masses or vaginal discharge, which become key elements of gynecological discourse in the following centuries.

In conclusion, Zhang's prescriptions and etiologies reflect a view of the female body as susceptible to vacuity and invasion by cold or wind, external pathogens which then impact the descent of menstrual blood and can lead to all sorts of associated symptoms. Beyond that, however, the female body is treated as identical with the male, with the exception of pregnancy and postpartum conditions, menstruation, and vaginal problems. Zhang himself states in the beginning of the *Jingui yaolüe* that "a physician of superior skills treats the root of disorders," subsequently qualifying that, "if cases of a chronic condition are aggravated by an acute condition, he should first treat the acute condition before treating the chronic condition."[22] But when it came to female bodies, it seems that women's underlying root pathologies were seen as too mysterious to be successfully treated by male physicians of Zhang's time. The early Chinese medical treatment of women was therefore apparently limited to the treatment of acute symptoms, without any attempt at diagnosing, much less treating, a root cause.

Lou wu se (Leaking in five colors): *The Zhubing yuanhou lun*

Several centuries later, Chao Yuanfang's 巢元方 *Zhubing yuanhou lun* 諸病源候論 (On the origins and symptoms of the various diseases),[23]

[22] Zhang, *Jingui yaolüe*, 1.20 and 43, respectively.

[23] Chao Yuanfang, *Zhubing yuanhou lun* (ca. 610; reprint, Beijing: Renmin weisheng chubanshe, 1992).

composed in the early seventh century, reflects a far more sophisticated and elaborate conception of the female body in both theory and practice. Being the first text to attempt a categorization of women's disorders, it laid the foundations for an emerging literature of special prescriptions and treatment methods to support and boost women's health. The innovative organization and theoretically informed etiologies express a view of the female body as endangered by reproduction, prone to vacuity and cold invasion, and therefore in need of special protection and attention. Out of eight *juan* on women's disorders, the first four are titled "the various symptoms of women's miscellaneous disorders," followed by four *juan* dealing with pregnancy, childbirth, and obstetrics. The miscellaneous chapters cover disorders considered as gendered because they are either specific to female anatomy, such as conditions of the female genitals or breasts, or because—and this addition is highly significant—they are seen as particularly common in women, such as wind stroke, digestive disorders, or abdominal masses. Of particular importance are here two subsections on what Chao considered the most central of all female disorders, leaking of a variety of fluids from the vagina, or, as one of the entry headings calls it, "leaking in five colors" (漏五色 *lou wu se*). These disorders are divided into menstrual problems and *daixia*, a term now used mostly in the technical sense of "vaginal discharge." In the discussion of *daixia* is found an essay that quotes a list of the so-called "thirty-six disorders which are mentioned in the various prescriptions [texts]." This is a classic list of women's disorders, found with little variation in numerous other texts.[24]

> What the various prescription [texts] call the Thirty-Six Disorders are namely the Twelve Concretions, the Nine Pains, the Seven Injuries, the Five Damages, and the Three Pathological Solidifications.
>
> The Twelve Concretions refer to the substance being discharged; the first one is like white lard; the second one like blue-green blood; the third one like purple juice; the fourth one like red flesh; the fifth one like scabby pus; the sixth one like bean juice; the seventh one like mallow broth; the eighth one like congealed blood; the ninth one like fresh, watery blood; the tenth one like rice-rinsing liquid; the eleventh one like menstrual blood; the twelfth one like menses at the wrong time.
>
> As for the Nine Pains, the first one is pain from injury to the inside of the genitals; the second, pain inside the genitals associated with inhibited and

[24] It is quoted, for example, in Sun, *Beiji qianjin yaofang*, 4.3.52-53, and in Tana Yasuyori 丹波康頼, ed., *Ishinpo* 醫心方 (982; reprint, Beijing: Huaxia chubanshe, 1996), 21.24.438.

dribbling urination; the third, pain accompanying urination; the fourth, pain from contracting cold; the fifth, abdominal pain at the onset of menstruation; the sixth, pain from *qi* fullness; the seventh, pain inside the genitals as if from gnawing bugs with liquid being discharged; the eighth, pulling pain below the flanks; the ninth, waist pain.

As for the Seven Injuries; the first one is injury from food; the second, injury from *qi*; the third, injury from cold; the fourth, injury from exertion; the fifth, injury from sex; the sixth, injury from pregnancy; and the seventh, injury from sleep.

As for the Five Damages; the first one is pain in the vagina; the second, pain from being struck by heat or cold; the third, tense and confined pain in the lower abdomen; the fourth, numbness of the internal organs; and the fifth, a crooked vagina with pain stretching to the back.

As for the Three Pathological Solidifications, the first one is obstructed and blocked menstrual flow, and the other two are not recorded.[25]

In neat numerical order, this list provides us with a comprehensive record of what were considered specifically female conditions in the seventh century.

A closer look at the etiologies for each disorder as they are covered in the individual enumerations of the text reveals further clues: First, the varieties of menstrual problems and vaginal discharge, as well as other disorders like abdominal masses, digestive disorders, and infertility, are explained with almost identical etiologies. All are associated with the root cause of taxation, which in turn is caused by childbirth. Having damaged *qi* and Blood, childbirth leads to physical vacuity, thereby making the body susceptible to an invasion by wind and/or cold, which lodge in the uterus. From there, cold causes Blood to congeal rather than to flow freely, while wind injures the channels responsible for the smooth movement of Blood. In both cases, this affects the monthly descent of Blood as menses, its gathering in the womb to nurture the fetus during pregnancy, or its ascent after childbirth into the breasts as breast milk. When *qi* is vacuous and therefore unable to control and restrain blood, this pathology can easily turn into vaginal discharge in the five colors when "the Blood in the channels is injured and therefore mixes with filthy fluids, forming vaginal discharge."[26] The color of the discharge provides important etiological clues about which internal organ is primarily affected. On the basis of correlative thinking and the association of the five colors with the five phases and five inter-

---

[25] Chao, *Zhubing yuanhou lun*, 38.50.1121-24.

[26] Chao, *Zhubing yuanhou lun*, 37.25.1093.

nal organs, green points to the liver, yellow to the spleen, red to the heart, white to the lungs, and black to the kidneys.

As mentioned above, the etiologies in the numerous subcategories are quite repetitive and therefore perhaps of little practical use. But it is still significant that the author devoted twenty-one separate entries, or almost four times as much space as for menstruation, to vaginal discharge. Overlooked or ignored in the previously discussed *Jingui yaolüe*, vaginal discharge came to be regarded by Chao as central to women's health. As a result, this pathology came to overshadow the other conditions that had originally been included under the term *daixia*, "below the girdle." In addition to its traditional use as a general term for women's conditions or a reference to the location of women's disorders "below the girdle," it had by Chao's times acquired the technical meaning of a specific gynecological pathology that was associated with the symptom of vaginal discharge. The most complete description of this pathology is found in the essay "Thirty-Six Symptoms of *Daixia*" translated above.

From the Tang period on, this topic was increasingly displaced by a focus on menstruation. What else but a deep concern for the vulnerability of the female body could have motivated an elite author and court physician like Chao to pay such attention to women's vaginal fluids, a substance which must have been quite appalling to a proper gentleman? His work therefore stands out not so much for the sophistication and creativity of his insights or for their practical applicability, but for his efforts to find the pathology at the root of women's health and to understand the female body in a systematic and theoretically grounded way.

Chao Yuanfang created or perpetuated a view of women's health as particularly susceptible and vulnerable because of their reproductive functions. Admittedly, the resulting malfunctions of the female body, rooted in and radiating outward from the mysterious area inside the lower abdomen called "*daixia*," remained inaccessible to the gaze of the male physician. Nevertheless, Chao raised the prospect of their consistent and rational interpretation and treatment through a highly specific diagnosis of a woman's discharge of pathological fluids from the vagina, the *yindao* 陰道 (*Yin* path) which led to these hidden regions. Related to this, Chao appears to be the first author to state the significance of women's menstrual and vaginal discharge for diagnosing underlying root patterns of systemic imbalances and weaknesses that were hidden inside women's bodies and ultimately led to infertility. He thereby laid the foundations for an aspect of gynecology which became increasingly central and sophisticated in later periods.

E lu (Noxious dew): The *Beiji qianjin yaofang*

Only decades after Chao Yuanfang's theoretical advances, Sun Simiao completed the *Beiji qianjin yaofang* 備急千金要方 (Essential prescriptions for every emergency worth a thousand pieces of gold) around 652 CE. In this groundbreaking medical encyclopedia of over five thousand entries, the three *juan* titled "prescriptions for women" form the first major section in the text, followed by pediatrics, general medicine, and, lastly, life-prolonging self-cultivation techniques. Sun Simiao is a key figure in the development of gynecology for being the first to stress the centrality of women's health for perpetuating the family lineage and to connect this with the individual practice of "nurturing life," *yangsheng* 養生. He is also the first author to explicitly state and justify the need for a literature of "separate prescriptions," *bie fang* 別方, for women.

This statement is found in a key passage in his famous introductory essay to the section on "prescriptions for women." I am quoting it here at length because of its elegance and succinctness, the complexity of ideas raised, and its subsequent significance for the history of gynecology.

> The reason for the existence of separate prescriptions for women is that they are different because of pregnancy, childbirth, and vaginal flooding. Therefore, women's disorders are ten times more difficult to treat than men's. In the classics, it is stated that "women are copious accumulations of *yin* and are constantly inhabited by dampness."[27]
>
> From the age of fourteen on, [a woman's] *yin qi* floats up and spills over, [causing] a hundred thoughts to pass through her heart. Internally, it damages the five organs; externally, it injures the disposition and complexion. The retention and discharge of menstrual fluids is alternately early or delayed, obstructed Blood lodges and congeals, and the central pathways are cut off. It is impossible to discuss the entirety of damages and fallout among these con-

[27] The origin of this quote is unclear. Given Sun's at least fragmentary familiarity with Indian medicine, it could be a translation from an Ayurvedic source because of its closeness to humoral theory. For the influence of Indian medicine on Sun Simiao, see several articles by Vijaya Deshpande, such as "Indian Influences on Early Chinese Ophthalmology: Glaucoma as a Case Study," *Bulletin of the School of Oriental and African Studies,* 62.2 (1999): 306-22.

> ditions. The raw and the cooked are deposited together,[28] vacuity and repletion alternate with each other, noxious Blood [leftover from childbirth] leaks internally, and the *qi* in the vessels is injured and exhausted... .
>
> In cases where seasonal *qi* has caused illness and where vacuity, repletion, cold, or heat have caused a problem, [women are to be treated] the same as men, the only exception being that, if they fall ill while carrying a fetus in pregnancy, toxic drugs must be avoided. In cases when their various disorders are identical to men's [conditions], knowledge of them can be obtained as they occur throughout the various volumes. Nevertheless, women's cravings and desires exceed men's, and they contract illness at twice the rate of men. In addition, they are imbued with affection and passion, love and hatred, envy and jealousy, and worry and rancor, which are lodged firmly in them. Since they are unable to control their emotions by themselves, the roots of their disorders are deep and it is difficult to obtain a cure in their treatment.[29]

Here, Sun Simiao constructs a multifaceted explanation for the medical need to recognize the female body as different. His discussion takes into consideration not only physiological factors, but also psychological and even cultural ones, all of which cause the medical treatment of women to be "ten times more difficult than men's." This essay is a powerful appeal to physicians' humanitarian duty to heal female bodies which are seen as particularly vulnerable for several reasons. Because of the stresses of pregnancy, childbirth, and resulting hemorrhaging, they are prone to vacuity, which could lead to any number of physical and psychological problems. In addition, women's excess of *yin qi* associated with sexual maturation causes emotional instability, damage to the internal organs, menstrual disorders, and problems with the flow of Blood and *qi* in the channels.

When we read the essay above in conjunction with the individual prescription entries that follow, the etiologies expressed by Sun Simiao reflect the notion, introduced in the earlier *Zhubing yuanhou lun* by Chao Yuanfang, that a vacuous female body, forced open in the process of childbirth, is liable to an invasion by cold and wind. Sneaking in through the vagina, these external pathogens can attack and block Blood and *qi* in the channels and from there wreak havoc in any of the internal organs for years to come. Moreover, it turns out that the most dangerous pathology for women, in Sun's eyes, is the lingering presence of a substance called *e lu* 惡露 (noxious dew). This evocative term refers to old Blood left over in the uterus after childbirth, the most common symptom of which is blocked menstru-

[28] Presumably a reference to digestive problems.
[29] Sun, *Beiji qianjin yaofang*, 2.1.14.

ation. It is considered extremely pathogenic and therefore has to be eliminated completely by means of numerous uterus-cleansing and Blood-dispersing prescriptions.

Associated with an endless list of symptoms not only inside the body for the rest of the woman's life, but also outside, *e lu* is feared as highly offensive to the spirits. To this day, a traditional Chinese woman's postpartum recovery is often covered by a host of taboos aimed at protecting her from premature contact with society and the natural environment. Postpartum taboos in the early gynecological literature express, on the one hand, the authors' paternalistic concern for the mother's extremely depleted and vulnerable physical state. On the other hand, though, the numerous references to magico-religious etiologies and treatments reflect a simultaneous awareness of the pathogenic powers of the Blood of childbirth and the risks of handling this substance. To cite just one example, in 1237, several centuries after the *Beiji qianjin yaofang*, Chen Ziming 陳自明 (ca. 1190-1270) compiled the *Furen daquan liangfang* 婦人大全良方 (All-inclusive good prescriptions for women). Particularly the section on childbirth contains a large percentage of religious treatments like invocations, talismans, astrological calculations, divinations, and various rituals to prevent offending the spirits during childbirth. Found in the lengthy discussion of postpartum taboos is even a strict warning that laundry that has been stained by childbirth must not be dried in the sunlight, or one will risk injury by evil spirits.[30]

To return to Sun Simiao's introductory essay, the effects of women's reproductive functions range from a general state of vacuity to specific conditions like emotional volatility during menstruation or the presence of rotting Blood in the uterus for years after childbirth. This underlying and often invisible vulnerability can then lead to severe injuries from fairly harmless secondary causes like an immoderate diet, sexual intercourse during menstruation or too soon after childbirth, or an invasion of wind by an innocent visit to the outhouse. After stressing that "women's cravings and desires exceed their husbands'… they contract illness at twice the rate of men and … because they are unable to control their emotions, the roots of

[30] Chen Ziming, *Furen daquan liangfang* (1237; reprint, Beijing: Renmin weisheng chubanshe, 1996), 18:1.487.

their disorders are deep," the essay concludes by emphasizing the importance of childbearing for society at large.

In the course of this argument, Sun first states that reproduction plays a central role in women's lives since "bearing children is the adult role in women's destiny and fate."[31] Going further, he even advises that "specialists in the art of nurturing life [*yangsheng zhi jia* 養生之家] should particularly instruct their sons and daughters to study these three *juan* of women's recipes until they comprehend them thoroughly" to prepare for any "harvests of unexpected surprises.." and "to prevent premature and wrongful death."[32] Even servants involved in childcare "cannot afford not to study them. Thus, they should routinely write out a copy and carry it on their person, clutched to their bosom, in order to guard against the unexpected."[33] The next essay states, "Marriage and childbearing are the basis of human affairs and the foundation of a king's transformative power. The sages set out the teachings and completely discussed their purport …"[34]

In a subtle but highly significant twist, Sun here extends the common elite practice of macrobiotic hygiene, i.e. physical cultivation with the purpose of prolonging one's life, to cover not only the practitioner's individual body but to also include past and, most importantly, future generations. The importance of female bodies in this context becomes immediately obvious, a fact that the ancient sages had already recognized. Protecting and preserving women's health was therefore an essential task for any elite gentleman, since it could, if neglected or ignored, result in potentially grave consequences for society as a whole. This respect for the female body was doubtlessly further strengthened by Sun Simiao's personal and active involvement as a Daoist priest and practitioner of religious cultivation. In stark contrast with the negative association of the female body with impurity, transgression, and material desire in Buddhism, it was celebrated in Daoism for its identification with *yin* as complementary to *yang*, and with motherhood and the ability to give and nurture life.

In order to round out our discussion of female pathology in the *Beiji qianjin yaofang*, a few words of caution are necessary. Its author,

[31] Sun, *Beiji qianjin yaofang*, 2.1.14.
[32] Sun, *Beiji qianjin yaofang*, 2.1.14.
[33] Sun, *Beiji qianjin yaofang*, 2.1.14.
[34] Sun, *Beiji qianjin yaofang*, 2.1.14.

Sun Simiao, might have been celebrated throughout China's history as the "King of Medicine" and as one of the founding fathers of Chinese medicine.[35] However, a careful study of contemporaneous biographical sources reveals that he was clearly not a professionally practicing physician as much as an elite polymath interested in pursuing the various connections between the macrocosm and such microcosms as the human body and the body politic with the ultimate purpose of "nurturing life."[36] As such, he was anything but a specialist in gynecology and probably limited his role mostly to collecting, transmitting, synthesizing, and preserving other people's practical experience. Lastly, the *Beiji qianjin yaofang* belongs to the medical genre of prescription literature. As such, it is directly oriented towards clinical application and mostly refrains from theoretical elaborations and explanations. While it has been quoted extensively ever since as the foundational text of gynecology, it is still centuries away from a consistent treatment of women based on a holistic understanding of the female body.

In spite of these limitations, the "prescriptions for women" in the *Beiji qianjin yaofang* reflect the care with which Sun Simiao constructed a justification for "prescriptions for women" as a separate medical category. The persuasive power of his arguments, exemplified by the lengthy passage translated above, is perhaps best illustrated by the fact that this text continues to be cited and discussed even in contemporary gynecological publications.[37] Sun's rationale for the gender-specific treatment of women has remained unchallenged to the present day. Moreover, Sun's passionate appeal to his elite readers to give precedence to women's health, on the dual basis of their

[35] See, for example, Paul U. Unschuld, *Medicine in China: Historical Artifacts and Images* (New York: Prestel Verlag, 2000), 88-95; Gan Zuwang 干祖望, *Sun Simiao pingzhuan* 孫思邈評傳 (Jiangsu: Nanjing daxue chubanshe, 1995); and the various articles found in "Jinian Sun Simiao shishi 1300 zhounian zhuanji" 紀念孫思邈逝世1300 週年專輯, *Zhonghua yishi zazhi* 中華醫史雜誌 13.1 (1983).

[36] See Nathan Sivin, *Chinese Alchemy: Preliminary Studies* (Cambridge, Mass.: Harvard University Press, 1968), 81-144; and Sabine Wilms, *The Female Body in Medieval Chinese Medicine: A Translation and Interpretation of the 'Prescriptions for Women' in Sun Simiao's* Bei ji qian jin yao fang" (Taos, NM: Paradigm Publications, forthcoming in 2005), Prolegomena, Chapter 2 .1, as well as the full translation of Sun Simiao's biography in the appendix.

[37] To give just two examples, see Luo Yuankai 羅元愷, chief ed., *Zhongyi fuke xue* 中醫婦科學 (Taipei: Zhiyin chubanshe, 1997); Zhang Qiwen 張奇文, ed., *Fuke zabing* 婦科雜病(Beijing: Renmin weisheng chubanshe, 1995).

central role in the perpetuation of the family and their weakness and vulnerability which resulted from this role, did not fall on deaf ears during his own times either. Gynecological theory and practice advanced rapidly in the centuries following the publication of the *Beiji qianjin yaofang* in a process that culminated in the publication of the above-mentioned *Furen daquan liangfang* in the late Song period.

Menstrual Balancing and the Formation of Gynecology in the Song Period

Sun Simiao built a convincing foundation, based on moral, social, medical, and, one could even claim, cosmological arguments, for the significance of healthy, that is, procreating, female bodies. During the Tang and Song periods, physicians responded to his call and developed the clinical experience and theoretical foundations to ensure the practical application of Sun's goals. According to Charlotte Furth, "In the Song dynasty, medical thought appeared more concerned with female difference than either earlier or later in Chinese history."[38] Promoted by the imperial court and supported by a Neo-Confucian ideology that encouraged an application and extension of the traditionally sanctioned fields of intellectual inquiry, gynecology thus became a respected field of medical specialization. A sophisticated medical literature about the female body was produced and disputed by male literati motivated by a humanitarian concern for the welfare of the state and its population. For these authors, the key to understanding the female body came to be found in the flow of female Blood, which in traditional Chinese medicine can manifest as menstrual fluid, breast milk, nourishment to the fetus in the womb, or even as congealed abdominal masses. Blood thus served as the key with which Song authors resolved the tension between an androgynous body of classical *yin-yang* theory and a living female body which functioned, suffered, and responded in distinctly female ways.

The recognition of Blood as the primary vital fluid in the female body constitutes a central medical innovation in the development of Chinese gynecology. The central role of blood for a body's health might not surprise a reader imbedded in a modern biomedical framework, in which this is one of the most obvious and un-

[38] Furth, *A Flourishing Yin*, 60-61.

disputable truths about the human body. But in the context of the early history of Chinese medicine, the association of women and blood marks a fascinating departure from an established orthodoxy based on the centrality not of blood, but of *qi*, the material basis and life-sustaining force of all existence. The discovery of *qi*—including its role within the body and between the inside and outside of the body, its movement in the vessels, and its treatment with exercise, diet, drugs, acupuncture, and other therapies—can be seen as perhaps the single most important development in the history of Chinese medicine. This notion of the centrality of *qi* has remained unchallenged, even in its modern confrontation and synthesis with biomedical medicine, in China as well as in the West. As Paul Unschuld pointed out in a recent study of the *Huangdi neijing*,

> … at some point during the early Han dynasty the diagnosis of disease through an assessment of the status of blood gave way to diagnosis by means of an interpretation of the *qi* movement in the vessels, and a treatment designed to let blood was replaced by an application of needles to influence the flow of *qi*. … [Consequently,] physiology and pathology and diagnosis and treatment were largely directed at manipulating the organism's *qi*.[39]

Ever since, Chinese medicine has been based on an androgynous human body that is diagnosed, explained, and treated on the basis of the state of *qi*. However, Chen Ziming, perhaps the greatest gynecological author of all times in China, argued in 1273: "When treating disease, the ancients first discussed that which they focused on. In men, one regulates *qi*. In women, one regulates Blood."[40] Moreover, in addition to its juxtaposition with male *qi* as the substance most essential for general health, female Blood was also seen by Chen as parallel to male *jing* 精 (essence) in the context of reproductive functions: "Men think of the bedroom when their essence is exuberant; women crave pregnancy when their Blood is exuberant."[41]

In diagnostic and therapeutic terms, the interest in female Blood was expressed by an increasing focus on menstruation as the outward expression of deeper and often hidden internal processes in the female body. Through the careful diagnosis of a woman's menstrual cycle, Song physicians managed to classify the complex di-

---

[39] Paul U. Unschuld, *Huang Di nei jing su wen: Nature, Knowledge, Imagery in an Ancient Chinese Medical Text* (Berkeley: University of California Press, 2003), 149.

[40] Chen, *Furen Daquan liangfang*, 6.9.174.

[41] Chen, *Furen Daquan liangfang*, 6.4.168.

versity of women's symptoms and signs into underlying diagnostic patterns of blood flow which directly pointed at treatment strategies to be applied (at least theoretically) in a systematic and consistent way. Rather than interpreting menstruation in terms of productivity as the absence of a fetus or a debilitating loss of vital substance, they associated the menstruating female body with the powerful cultural ideals of regularity on the one hand, and uninterrupted flow on the other.

The Rise of Menstruation in the Organization and Etiologies of "Prescriptions for Women"

Given the importance of Blood and menstruation in Chinese gynecology from the Song period on, allow me to retrace the development of this view. Even a cursory survey of the organization and content of the "prescriptions for women" reveals a gradual shift in the understanding of female pathology. The following paragraphs are based on a content analysis of the major medical texts on women's health from the Han to Song periods, including the three texts discussed above and concluding with the already quoted *Furen daquan liangfang* by Chen Ziming.[42] For the purposes of this article, I subdivided the contents of each text into the categories of reproduction, menstruation, vaginal discharge, and miscellaneous conditions. In this, I have followed the organization employed most commonly in the primary sources themselves.[43]

---

[42] In addition, it considers the *Waitai miyao* 外台秘要 by Wang Xi 王熹 (752), the *Ishinpo*, the *Taiping sheng hui fang* 太平聖惠方 by Wang Huaiyin 王懷隱, chief ed. (978-992; reprint, Beijing: Renmin weisheng chubanshe, 1982), and the *Nüke baiwen* 女科百問 by Qi Zhongfu 齊仲甫 (1220; reprinted in *Zhenben yishu jicheng* 珍本醫書集成, vol. 8, *fuke lei* 婦科類 (Shanghai: Shanghai kexue jishu chubanshe, 1985), 1047-93).

[43] Most received primary sources from the pre-Song period are accessible to us only in editions that could have been altered and modified quite a bit by their Song editors. I am aware that the practice of classifying entries into categories that were to a certain extent conceived as separate only from the Song period onward is fraught with many dangers. However, for the purpose of indicating general trends, it is possible to categorize prescriptions and symptoms according to titles, location in the text, lists of indications, and intended drug actions. Moreover, in the case of Sun Simiao's *Beiji qianjin yaofang*, a comparison of the received text with manuscripts and fragments pre-dating the Song modifications has failed to reveal such major discrepancies as to invalidate my methodology.

The topics directly related to reproduction, namely fertility, pregnancy, obstetrics, postpartum care, and lactation, are of less concern here because they are obviously gendered and, moreover, their proportion remained basically consistent during the time period under consideration.[44] Their relative size varies mostly depending on the extent to which they included advice related to midwifery and magical, shamanistic, and religious material, such as placenta burial, astrological taboos, fetal education (that is, attempts to manipulate the fetus's gender, fate, and personality during pregnancy), and childbirth rituals. Nevertheless, they always constitute between half and three quarters of the text as a whole. Religious treatments and midwifery were apparently regarded as marginal or inappropriate for the interest of elite medical practitioners by some authors, included by others in some detail for the sake of comprehensiveness, or referred to as being located in other categories of technical literature. Their presence or absence in a text is therefore related more to a particular author's background, interests, and intention, than the date of its composition. The topic of "miscellaneous conditions" served as a grab-bag for all other disorders regarded as gendered by the authors, from vaginal and mammary problems to wind stroke and dreams of intercourse with ghosts. The chart below tracks the relative proportions of entries related to menstruation and vaginal discharge in texts from the late Han to the Song period. It includes data from the following texts, marked by their approximate date of composition and arranged in chronological order: *Jingui yaolüe*, *Zhubing yuanhou lun*, *Beiji qianjin yaofang*, *Waitai miyao* 外台秘要 (Essential secrets of the Palace Library, 752), *Ishinpo* 醫心方 (Prescriptions at the heart of medicine, 982), *Taiping sheng hui fang* 太平聖惠方 (Imperial Grace formulary, 992), *Nüke baiwen* 女科百問 (One hundred questions on gynecology, 1220), and *Furen daquan liangfang* 婦人大全良方 (1237).

[44] For more information on reproduction in early Chinese medicine, see Lee Jen-der 李貞德, "Han Tang zhijian qiuzi yifang shitan – jian lun fuke lanshang yu xingbie lunshu" 漢唐之間求子醫方試探—兼論婦科濫觴與性別論述, *Bulletin of the Institute of History and Sinology, Academia Sinica* 中央研究院歷史語言研究所集刊 68.2 (1997):283-367, as well as her "Han Tang zhijian yishu zhong de shengchan zhi dao" 漢唐之間醫書中的生產之道 *Bulletin of the Institute of History and Sinology, Academia Sinica* 67.3 (1996):533-654.

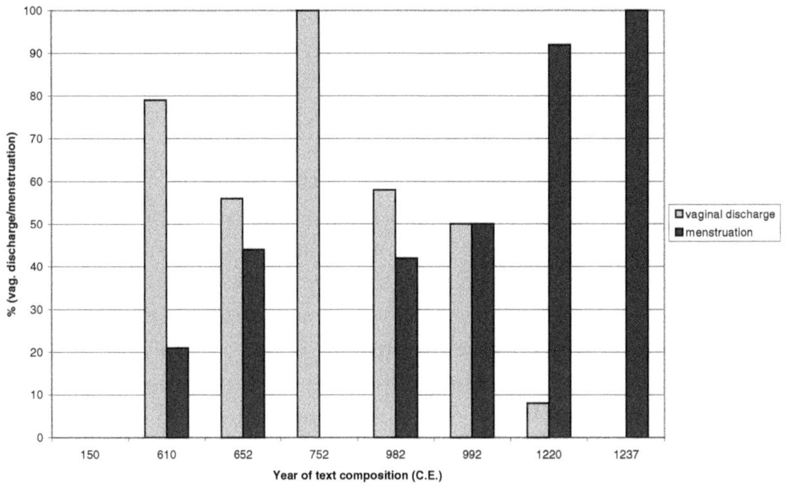

Proportion of Vaginal Discharge and Menstruation in "Prescriptions for Women," Han to Song Periods

The earliest text in the medical literature with a separate section on women, Zhang Ji's *Jingui yaolüe,* discussed above, refers to all women's conditions as *daixia* in its most literal sense of "below the girdle." It lacks any attempt at categorizing or systematically approaching female conditions and contains no mention or recognition of the pathology of vaginal discharge. Interrupted menstruation is only mentioned in passing as a symptom. However, it is noteworthy that in several instances the location of women's disorders is referred to as *xueshi* (Blood chamber), thus already indicating a relationship between specifically female pathologies and Blood.

Looking at the following texts from the seventh and eighth centuries, the advances made in terms of diagnosis and treatment are striking. In the earliest of these, namely Chao Yuanfang's *Zhubing yuanhou lun,* menstrual disorders, vaginal discharge, abdominal masses, and infertility are treated in separate categories, but explained with virtually identical etiologies. *Daixia* in the specific meaning of "vaginal discharge" stands out not only for being the single largest disease category with numerous subcategories, but also for being the basis for at least relating to most other symptoms and therefore for being instrumental in shaping Chao's ideas about female pathology in general.

A similar overlap and confusion between categories can be witnessed in Sun Simiao's *Beiji qianjin yaofang*. When we read Sun's "prescriptions for women" as a whole, the restoration of a regular and healthy blood flow, particularly as it relates to proper postpartum care, emerges as the greatest concern and perhaps the most prevalent underlying theme in Sun's treatment of female bodies. After the first *juan* on fertility, pregnancy, obstetrics, and lactation, the treatment of postpartum conditions, comprising almost the entire second *juan*, constitutes the largest single section or almost one third of the entire text. As the choice of medicinals and the lists of symptoms suggest, the prescriptions found here have two major goals, namely the supplementation of a body depleted by pregnancy, childbirth, and lactation, and the complete elimination of *e lu*, stale blood left over in the womb after childbirth. They are intended not to stop postpartum bleeding, but, on the contrary, to encourage a profuse blood flow after childbirth, a necessary condition for the elimination of *e lu* and for eventually resuming a regular menstrual period.

Even in cases of extreme hemorrhaging or chronic bleeding after childbirth, blood-stopping medicinals are to be avoided: "In the treatment of incessant leaking of blood, maybe caused by recent damage to the fetus [that is, bleeding during the pregnancy] or the fact that the residual blood after childbirth has not dispersed but become solidified, preventing the entrance to the uterus from closing and causing dribbling and dripping blood loss for several days or months without stopping, one may not yet use the various decoctions for interrupting the blood flow. ... When the solidified blood has been dispersed, then the dribbling and dripping bleeding will stop on its own [since it is] also gradually being transformed, dispersed, and reduced."[45]

Indicating the long-ranging significance of the etiology of incomplete elimination of postpartum blood, this statement is found not in the postpartum section in the second *juan*, but in the section on *daixia* in the third *juan*. This last *juan* is divided into the three major topics of "supplementing and boosting," blocked and irregular menstruation, and vaginal discharge. Throughout the third *juan*, both vaginal discharge and menstrual problems are constantly linked to each other and to the presence of *e lu* as related, parallel, and often overlapping symptoms. They both indicate an underlying vacuity and weakness of blood and *qi*, resulting from women's reproductive

---

[45] Sun, *Beiji qianjin yaofang*, 4.3.56.

functions. As the logical treatment for any of these symptoms, the prescriptions include a sizable component of stabilizing and supplementing drugs like *yuyuliang* 禹餘糧 (limonite), *longgu* 龍骨 (dragon bone), *renshen* 人參 (ginseng), *lurong* 鹿茸 (velvet deer antler), *danggui* 當歸 (Chinese angelica), and *shaoyao* 芍藥 (white peony), on the one hand, and of blood-moving and pathogen-expelling drugs like *taoren* 桃仁 (peach pit), *dahuang* 大黃 (rhubarb), *shuizhi* 水蛭 (leech), *mengchong* 虻蟲 (horse fly), *xixin* 細辛 (asarum), and *chaihu* 柴胡 (bupleurum), on the other.

The following prescription for "Dried Ginger Pills" from the chapter on "stopped menstrual flow" will give readers a taste of the diagnostic specificity and sensitivity to women's health problems reflected in Sun's text. It also serves to demonstrate the above-mentioned etiological links and therapeutic goals:

> Dried Ginger Pills
> For treating women [who suffer from] emaciation with chills and fevers; soreness and wasting disorder; inertia and sluggishness; propping fullness in the chest; heaviness and pain in the shoulders, back, and spine; hardness, fullness, and accumulations in the abdomen, potentially with unbearable pain from the waist to the lower abdomen; vexation and aching in the four limbs; reverse flow in the hands and feet, cold reaching the elbows and knees, or with vexing fullness and vacuity heat in the hands and feet so that she feels like tossing herself into water; extreme pain in the hundred joints; constant discomfort and suspension pain below the heart; alternating chills and fevers; nausea, profuse drooling, and salivating every time in response to salty, sour, sweet, or bitter substances; or [an appearance of] the body like chicken skin; stopped menstrual flow; discomfort and difficulty with urination and defecation; eating without generating muscles:
>
> One *liang* 兩[46] each of *gan jiang* 乾薑 [dried ginger], *xiongqiong* 芎藭 [ligusticum wallichii], *fuling* 茯苓 [poria], *xiaoshi* 硝石 [niter], *xingren* 杏仁 [apricot pit], *shuizhi* 水蛭 [leech], *mengchong* 虻蟲 [horse fly], *taoren* 桃仁 [peach pit], *qicao* 蠐螬 [black chafer larva], and *zhechong* 蟅蟲 [wingless cockroach].
> Two *liang* each of *chaihu* 柴胡 [bupleurum], *shaoyao* 芍藥 [white peony], *renshen* 人參 [ginseng], *dahuang* 大黃 [rhubarb], *shujiao* 蜀椒 [zanthoxylum], and *danggui* 當歸 [Chinese angelica].
>
> Pulverize the sixteen ingredients above and mix them with honey into pills the size of parasol tree seeds. On an empty stomach, take three pills with fluid

[46] A measurement for medicinal ingredients. The *xiaoliang* 小兩 (small *liang*) which was supposed to be the standard for medicinal preparations during the Tang dynasty, averaged about 14 grams, according to archaeological evidence. See Qiu Guangming 丘光明, ed., *Zhongguo kexue jishu shi* 中國科學技術史: *Du liang heng juan* 度量衡卷 (Beijing: Kexue chubanshe, 2001), 336.

> [three times a day]. If no effect is noticed, increase the dosage to a maximum of ten pills [per dose].[47]

In contemporaneous materia medica literature, the medicinal ingredients chosen here had the intended effects of moving Blood, raising the body temperature, and supplementing Blood.[48] Thus, the prescription was intended to treat a condition caused by a combination of pathologies related to an impeded flow of Blood, a lowered body temperature, and Blood vacuity. This constellation of etiologies, in conjunction with the secondary symptoms found in the list of indications, suggests the same complex of ideas about female pathology that Chao Yuanfang had previously treated primarily under the category of vaginal discharge. What is new in Sun's prescriptions is the emphasis on a root pathology of blocked blood, especially after childbirth, and related to this, on its treatment by restoring and adjusting menstruation.

We can see an interpretation of women's bleeding emerging that is, to be sure, still influenced by ideas about its weakening and destabilizing effect on the female body. However, this negative view is increasingly replaced by a positive appreciation of female bleeding as a natural and healthy function, instrumental in ensuring reproductive health through the periodic emptying and cleansing of the uterus. Even more evocative is the equation of menstruation with a healthy movement and transformation of bodily fluids, with a proper balance, harmony, and mutual support between *qi* and blood, and with a regular discharge of the byproducts of women's reproductive functions. Rather than focusing on the weakening effects of this process, the central paradigm of female pathology becomes the lack of flow, reflected in expressions like *jingbi* 經閉 (blocked menstruation) or, even more suggestive, *yuejing bu tong* 月經不通 (a menstrual period that fails to penetrate/flow through). Subsequently, the primary cause of infertility was not found in the weakening effects of regular blood loss, but in its opposite, the retention of blood which, when failing to be released through its proper opening, formed blockages

---

47 Sun, *Beiji qianjin yaofang*, 41.2.49.

48 Namely the *Shennong bencao jing* 神農本草經 (Shennong's classic of materia medica) from the late Han period, which was edited, annotated, and enlarged by Tao Hongjing in the early sixth century. No academic translation is available in English. A good critical edition is Ma Jixing 馬繼興, ed., *Shennong bencao jing jizhu* 神農本草經輯注 (Beijing: Renmin weisheng chubanshe, 1995).

and abdominal masses, or ascended to the upper part of the body instead.

Menstruation in Song Gynecology

This interpretation of female Blood and menstruation became the hallmark of gynecology when it emerged in the Song dynasty as a respected medical specialty, to be practiced not only by such marginal, and probably most often illiterate, figures as midwives, shamans, or herbalists, but also by dedicated literati physicians who recognized the significance of the female body for the health of Chinese society at large. In the above chart, we can see a shift, between the Han and the Song periods, from vaginal discharge to menstruation as the most important pathology in light of which physicians approached both the diagnosis and treatment of the female body.

Already in the *Taiping sheng hui fang*, compiled by a team of court-appointed doctors in the tenth century, a new conception of gynecological disorders is obvious in the sections on "prescriptions for women" (*juan* 69-81 out of 100). Much of the actual content is copied from the previous literature, but it is rearranged and explained in light of a new theoretical foundation for interpreting women's bodies as gendered. The innovative organization of the text into chapters on wind stroke, vacuity taxation, aggregations and blood clots, menstruation, and vaginal discharge, followed by sections on pregnancy, childbirth, and postpartum treatments, illustrates a much advanced conception of women's health and illness. As we have already seen in earlier literature, women are in this text also characterized as plagued by a vacuity of Blood and *qi*. This is stated authoritatively in the introductory essay of the first section on wind stroke: "The fact that women suffer from vacuous and injured *qi* and Blood causes them to [suffer from] wind stroke."[49]

On a deeper level, the second *juan*, on "Supplementing Treatments for Women's Vacuity Injury," relates this vacuity to a root pathology of an imbalance of *qi* and Blood (*qi xue butiao* 氣血不調), in a subtle reformulation of Sun Simiao's famous introductory essay translated above: "The reason why separate prescriptions have been established for women is that their *qi* and blood are imbalanced. This

[49] Wang Huaiyin, *Taiping sheng hui fang*, 69.1.

is caused by their difference in terms of pregnancy, childbirth, and hemorrhaging damage." Further on, vacuity is interpreted as a secondary etiology: "When taxation damages *qi* and Blood, it causes vacuity injury. Then, wind and cold exploit the vacuity and attack." In their respective chapters, menstruation and vaginal discharge are explained in related and overlapping etiologies. Taxation damage causes a vacuity of the body, allowing wind to enter and congeal the Blood in the channels with the result of inhibited or stopped menstruation. Alternately, the *qi* in the thoroughfare vessel *chongmai* 衝脈 and controlling vessel *renmai* 任脈, when injured by taxation, becomes vacuous and therefore unable to control and restrain the flow of Blood in the channels. In that case, it flows out below as red vaginal discharge or pathological bleeding, instead of turning into breast milk during lactation, nurturing the fetus during pregnancy, or being discharged regularly as menstrual fluid.[50] The section related directly to menstruation comprises, strictly speaking, only six percent of the total text. But given the above-mentioned etiological connections and the obvious role of Blood in all reproductive disorders, the regulation and supplementation of Blood is clearly the most consistent therapeutic goal found in this text.

Only decades later, in 1220, Qi Zhongfu, a professor in the Imperial Medical Bureau, composed the *Nüke baiwen*. As Furth has stated, "it may well have been the first book to address gynecology on an equal basis with the gestational issues of pregnancy and postpartum."[51] In contrast to the *Taiping sheng hui fang* in which the section on "prescriptions for women" is limited strictly to conditions with clearly female-specific etiologies and therapies, the *Nüke baiwen* is a free-standing text dedicated exclusively to women's health, with a much more diverse content. Of its 100 questions, the first half concerns general ideas about women (1-5), menstruation (6-13), miscellaneous conditions (14-48) and two questions on vaginal discharge (49-50), while the second half covers pregnancy, obstetrics, and postpartum care. Menstruation constitutes almost one quarter of the content not directly related to reproduction, compared with a mere two percent for vaginal discharge and three quarters for miscellaneous conditions. Probably because the text was intended as a quick reference guide for questions on women's health, about half the topics in

[50] Wang, *Taiping sheng hui fang*, introductory essays, 72.1 and 73.1.
[51] Furth, *A Flourishing Yin*, 70.

the miscellaneous section, such as insanity, hair loss, jaundice, waist pain, body itch, and constipation, are not gender-specific at all, but were presumably included because of their prevalence in women. To give just one example of its medical advances, question six stresses the importance of differentiating between *yin* and *yang* conditions when diagnosing and treating menstrual problems. *Yin* conditions are characterized by a prevalence of cold which causes an impediment of flow and results in deficient and/or late menstrual periods, while *yang* conditions are linked to the presence of warmth, an excess flow, and early or excessive menstrual periods.[52] Similar to the earlier texts discussed above, the most common etiology is one of blood and *qi* disharmony, and blood vacuity and congestion, which facilitate an invasion of wind, a blockage in the channels, and subsequent inhibition of the menstrual flow.

The last, but definitely not least important text which concludes this brief survey of early Chinese gynecological literature is the *Furen daquan liangfang*. Chen Ziming, an experienced physician from a prestigious medical lineage, composed it in 1237 in order to synthesize his personal experience, his secret family prescriptions, and over forty gynecological texts, dating mostly from the Song dynasty. Confidently expressing pride in his professional specialization, he states in the introduction: "Now, the art of medicine is difficult. Medicine [as applied to] women is particularly difficult. And medicine in the midst of childbirth involves several bodies and is therefore yet more risky and difficult."[53] Long essays, like the one introducing the first major section on menstruation, demonstrate that, while ostensibly grounded in the literature of previous centuries, Song gynecology had become a rapidly advancing medical specialty. Chen's book represents the achievements of a life-long professional involvement in women's healthcare, incorporating both clinical experience and literary proficiency. Similar to the *Hundred Questions*, the importance of menstruation as the foundation for women's health is again expressed in the placement of the section on menstrual balancing, *yuetiao* 月調, at the very beginning of the text. It constitutes about eight percent of the total text, or twenty percent of the section that is not directly related to reproduction. The condition of vaginal discharge has by now become so insignificant that it is completely in-

[52] Qi Zhongfu, *Nüke baiwen*, 1052.
[53] Chen, *Furen daquan liangfang*, preface, i.

corporated into the category of menstruation as merely one of many symptoms which point toward root pathologies related to the flow of female Blood.

The discovery of menstruation as the key to women's health provided Song gynecologists with a theoretical foundation from which to understand the invisible processes inside women's bodies. They were thus able to consistently group women's symptoms into root patterns which pointed at effective and proven treatment strategies. From the tentative beginnings under such terms as "thirty-six diseases" or "*daixia*" and a concern with the dangers of women's loss of bodily fluids as blood and vaginal discharge, the medical literature expresses an ever-growing confidence in the ability of male literati physicians to detect, diagnose, and treat women's disorders. Most importantly, by establishing, restoring, and supporting a healthy and regular menstrual flow, they were finally able to actively treat and prevent the dreaded chronic conditions that so often threatened women's reproductive capacities and lives.

Conclusion: The Gendered Body Revisited

> "If the lord hadn't a knowd that the woman was gonna be stronger, he wouldn't a had the woman have the periods and the babies. Can you see a man having a baby?"[54]

We will never know whether some or any women in post-Han China could have related to this sentiment. Uttered by a retired homemaker from Baltimore in the 1980s, it should nevertheless make us question the unanimous acceptance of scientific paradigms, particularly if we contrast it with the dominant biomedical discourse on the debilitating effects of menstruation and childbirth and of women as the "weaker sex." The analysis above has centered on the paradigm by which the authors of "prescriptions for women" in post-Han imperial China interpreted the female body, based on their clinical experiences as well as their theoretical insights. To conclude this article, let us now return to the questions posed in the introduction, especially the last one regarding the relationship between male and female bodies.

---

[54] Phyllis Hood, in Emily Martin, *The Woman in the Body: A Cultural Analysis of Reproduction* (Boston: Beacon Press, 1987), 194.

The above discussion has revealed two different paradigms through which the male authors of early Chinese medical literature conceptualized this relationship. On the one hand, the early theoretical classics express a view of female and male bodies as homologous and equally close to an ideal sexually neutral human body, which, in its shifting balance of *yin* and *yang* attributes, served as a model for the universe and generative processes at large. While obviously informed by this literature, texts on "prescriptions for women" between the Han and Song periods gradually developed an alternative interpretation of the female body as categorically different from the male. Reproduction, the foundation of women's social role, threatened and weakened its health, necessitating gender-specific treatments. Women's sickness and health, diagnosis and treatment, all centered on the notion of Blood as a life-sustaining fluid that was, in a healthy body, distributed throughout and discharged from the body in regular, predictable rhythms. This uniquely female function was precisely what facilitated conception, pregnancy, childbirth, and lactation in the female body. Male physicians who specialized in the treatment of women perceived themselves as assisting in this natural process primarily by supporting, correcting, and promoting the flow of female Blood.

The recognition that the female body was categorically different from the male, initiated perhaps by Sun Simiao's statement about the need for "separate prescriptions for women," clearly conflicted with the idealized androgynous body depicted in the early classics. The development of gynecological literature over the following centuries is therefore a case of medical innovation, a topic that is generally associated more with the rapid pace of change in modern biomedical science than with Chinese medicine. As a collection of articles entitled *Innovation in Chinese Medicine* demonstrated a few years ago, however, the association of Chinese medicine with "traditional therapies and ancient practices which have been in place, unchanging, since time immemorial" has clearly been proven wrong.[55] While change occurs in any medical tradition, it can be interpreted and expressed in many different ways.

Laqueur's research on the history of sex in early Europe indicated that Western conceptions of the female body shifted dramatically in

---

[55] Elisabeth Hsu, ed., *Innovation in Chinese Medicine* (Cambridge: Cambridge University Press, 2001). Quotation from back cover jacket.

early modern Europe.[56] The earlier "one sex" model, derived from such Greek writers as Aristotle and Galen, viewed the sexes in a hierarchical but continuous relationship, determined by the amount of heat in the body, with the male as the ideal and the female as a less perfect replica. Since the female body contained less heat than the male, its reproductive organs were kept warm and protected on the inside of the body, but were otherwise homologous in the strict biological sense of that term, that is, "based upon their descent from a common evolutionary ancestor ... similar to each other in construction but ... modified to perform different functions, [like a] a bat's wing and a whale's flipper."[57] Since early European gynecology took the male body as the norm and defined the female body as a deviation therefrom, the uterus—*hystera* in Greek—became the key to understanding female pathology. The uterus was believed to become uncontrollable when not kept in place by regular pregnancies and to roam around in the body, causing all sorts of curious behavioral abnormalities that were subsumed under the condition of *hysteria*. As Plato stated, "The womb is an animal which longs to generate children. When it remains barren for too long after puberty, it is distressed and sorely disturbed, and straying about in the body and cutting off the passages of the breath, it impedes respiration and brings the sufferer into the extremist anguish and provokes all manner of diseases besides."[58]

In the wake of larger societal and economic changes in early modern Europe, both promoters of women's subordination as well as of their liberation constructed and supported a radical new model of incommensurability and biological divergence between the sexes. The growth of biological essentialism from the eighteenth century on further emphasized the importance of anatomical features, leading to a "two-sex" model of fundamental difference by reducing their relationship to the objective and absolute anatomical and physiological differences between male and female bodies. This "two-sex" model has been alternately criticized and encouraged by both feminists and anti-feminists, depending on their political agenda. But it remains the

[56] Thomas Laqueur, *Making Sex: Body and Gender from the Greeks to Freud* (Cambridge, Mass.: Harvard University Press, 1990).

[57] "Homology." *Encyclopædia Britannica Online*. 2004. <http://search.eb.com/eb?article?eu=41805> (accessed July 1, 2004).

[58] Plato, *Timaeus*. Trans. in Mark S. Micale, *Approaching Hysteria: Disease and its Interpretations* (Princeton, N.J.: Princeton University Press, 1995), 19.

most common way in which contemporary Western culture views male and female bodies and constructs gender difference.

In the Chinese case, the independent existence, propagation, and clinical efficacy of "separate prescriptions" for women forced medical theorists to refine their model of the human body and to accommodate the clinical reality of the female body into their reasoning in order to ensure its health and safety. In the European case, scientific theories and intellectual developments propelled the medical community to revise its "one-sex" model of an ideal male body and to conceptualize a female body as categorically different. In China, the ideal body of androgyny, which we might call a "dual-sex" body, was never challenged by gynecological theories stressing the uniqueness of female reproductive processes. As in other medical fields, Song gynecological advances simply added one more layer of sophistication and refinement to a tradition firmly rooted in the mystical insights of ancient sages. Thus it was possible to integrate the distinctly female body of Song gynecology into an overarching paradigm of androgyny that continued to emphasize the complementarity and homology of the sexes.

CHILDBIRTH IN EARLY IMPERIAL CHINA*

BY

JEN-DER LEE
(Institute of History and Philology, Academia Sinica)
(English translation by Sabine Wilms)

Abstract

By the eighth century, medical texts had come to agree that an expecting mother should take herbal medicine in the last month of pregnancy to ensure a quick and safe delivery. Delivery charts, previously separated for different purposes, were integrated into one chart with twelve sub-charts for each month of the year. Women usually took vertical positions during delivery and were most likely supported under the arms by midwives. Ritual techniques and manual manipulations were applied to solve complications such as breech birth. The former often implied resonant relations between the baby, its mother and her husband, while the latter sometimes elicited criticism from male doctors as unnecessary interventions. The new mother would be restrained from social contact in the first month after delivery, because of both her need to rest and the fear of pollution. Friends and relatives, however, would bring over precious and nutritious food to "nourish her body," said the medical texts, "not just to celebrate the child."

Introduction

Procreation played a central role in women's lives, and childbirth can be said to have been a crisis of life or death for pregnant women. If a pregnancy was successful, not only was the mother safe, but she also provided the household with descendants and labor. A smooth delivery was, as far as the family and community were concerned, a reason for celebration, as well as, for the participants and

* This article first appeared in Chinese in the *Bulletin of the Institute of History and Philology, Academia Sinica* 67.3 (1996): 533-642. The English translation was done by Dr. Sabine Wilms and revised by the author to incorporate current research. The Appendix from the original Chinese version, containing herbal recipes for treating complications and for postpartum care, is integrated into the main text in the English version.

helpers, an affirmation of their abilities and efforts. In the case of failure, the situation was entirely different. If the mother died and the child survived, the newborn child lost a mother, the household lost the mistress of the house, the situation of the surviving child became precarious, and poor families might have even lost their base of support. If the mother survived and the child died, then this failure at the last moment, after having nurtured the fetus for ten months, had an enormous impact on the parturient woman's body and mind.[1] A fetus that died in the womb, moreover, impacted the mother's safety. And if both mother and child died, then the family and community were most likely grief-stricken, and it was hard for the birth attendants to avoid incurring blame.

Birth is the stage at which the mother and the fetus separate after ten months of pregnancy, and, in terms of the biological phenomenon, there is little difference between the past and the present, China and the outside world. But the medical management, rituals and taboos, and ideas and concepts surrounding this stage can nevertheless vary according to the culture of the times. Thus, the circumstances of delivery in traditional Chinese society are well worth a thorough inquiry. Whether because searching for and gathering records is difficult, or whether scholars' interest has yet to be stimulated, up to now monographs about traditional childbirth rituals and gynecological and obstetrical medicine are rare. Moreover, detailed studies of childbirth culture concentrate mostly on developments in the late imperial period. Research studies on the situation in early imperial China are comparatively few.[2]

---

[1] Although gestation is considered to be nine months in the West, traditional Chinese perceived it as to have been ten months. Even today, in popular language, people still use "ten months of pregnancy" (*huaitai shiyue* 懷胎十月) to describe a woman's gestation pesiod.

[2] Guo Licheng 郭立誠, *Zhongguo shengyu lisu kao* 中國生育禮俗考 (Taipei: Wenshizhe chubanshe, 1971), is probably the earliest work on this subject. It describes the childbirth culture of traditional society, including praying for a son, fetal education, and all other aspects of childbirth rituals. Ma Dazheng 馬大正, *Zhongguo fuchanke fazhanshi* 中國婦產科發展史 (Shanxi: Kexue jiaoyu chubanshe, 1991), summarizes the development of Chinese gynecological and obstetrical science from pre-Qin (221-207 BCE) to the Republican period. Zhang Zhibin 張志斌, *Gudai Zhongyi fuchanke jibingshi* 古代中醫婦產科疾病史 (Beijing: Zhongyi guji chubanshe, 2000), is the most recent general history on gynecological and obstetrical disorders and includes discussions on childbirth complications. See the review [infra]. For discussions of specific periods, such as Patricia Ebrey's description of the abilities of people in the Song dynasty (960-

When researching the issue of infant abandonment in early imperial China, I realized that, following maternal death in childbirth, poor families had no choice but to consider abandoning the newborn. Therefore I wonder whether the many instances of infant abandonment at that time might not suggest the frequent occurrence of maternal death in childbirth?[3] Moreover, in my research on women's lives in early imperial China, I found that women married mostly between the ages of fourteen and eighteen, and the statistics on women's lifespans revealed that women's death rate peaked between the ages of twenty and thirty. This seems to suggest that childbirth-related conditions might have been one of the major causes of death for women at that time.[4] In ancient times, methods of birth control and abortion were not sufficiently refined and widespread, which

---

1279) to care for women in childbirth, see Ebrey, *The Inner Quarters: Marriage and the Lives of Chinese Women in the Song Period* (Berkeley: University of California Press, 1993), 172-76. Xiong Bingzhen (Ping-chen Hsiung) 熊秉真, in her examination of pediatric medicine in late imperial China, also touches upon the issues of childbirth care. See Xiong Bingzhen 熊秉真, *Youyou: chuantong zhongguo de qiangbao zhidao* 幼幼—傳統中國的襁褓之道 (Taipei: Lianjing chubangongsi, 1995), 53-102. Charlotte Furth's inspiring accounts describe the changes and continuities in gestation and birth from the Song to the late imperial period; Charlotte Furth, *A Flourishing Yin: Gender in China's Medical History, 960-1665* (Berkeley: University of California Press, 1999), 94-133, 134-54; and more recently, Yi-Li Wu, "Ghost Fetuses, False Pregnancies, and the Parameters of Medical Uncertainty in Classical Chinese Gynecology," *Nan Nü: Men, Women and Gender in Early and Imperial China* 4.2 (2002): 170-206. Only a few studies deal with the earlier periods, e.g., Li Jianmin 李建民, "Mawangdui Hanmu boshu 'Yuzang maibao tu' jianzheng" 馬王堆漢墓帛書禹藏埋胞圖箋證, *Bulletin of the Institute of History and Philology, Academia Sinica* 中央研究院歷史語言研究所集刊 65.4 (1994): 725-832. Li's article discusses placenta burial customs and rituals as well as the idea of correspondence between Heaven and the human world in early China. But Li's article, like Xiong's book, concentrates on the survival and growth of the newborn and relatively seldom touches on the childbearing woman. My article on wet nurses also touches upon postpartum care; see Jen-der Lee, "Wet Nurses in Early Imperial China," *Nan Nü:* 2.1 (2000): 1-39. A more recent study by Sabine Wilms on women's medicine and its manifestations on the female body discusses the medicinal and cultural significance of childbirth to some extent. See Wilms, "The Female Body in Medieval Chinese Medicine: A Translation and Interpretation of the 'Women's Recipes' in Sun Simiao's *Beiji qianjin yaofang*," (Ph.D. diss., University of Arizona, 2002), 59-84.

[3] Li Zhende (Jen-der Lee) 李貞德, "Han Sui zhijian de 'shengzi buju' wenti" 漢隋之間的生子不舉問題, *Bulletin of the Institute of History and Philology, Academia Sinica* 66.3 (1995): 747-812.

[4] Jen-der Lee, "The Life of Women in the Six Dynasties," *Journal of Women and Gender Studies* 婦女與兩性學刊 4 (1993): 47-80, Tables I, V.

increased women's chances of pregnancy.[5] If a woman married at age fourteen, stopped menstruating at forty-nine, and gave birth to ten children, she was involved in childrearing for most of her adult years, giving birth approximately once every three years. Since besides delivering her own children, a woman also observed, discussed, and assisted in the deliveries of her female friends' and relatives' children, birth was a common experience in most women's lives.

Reproduction also influenced women's physical and emotional health. In the view of the Liu-Song (420-79) doctor Chen Yanzhi 陳延之, among women who marry and undergo childbirth too early, "the root of the kidneys has not yet been established, and birth then injures the kidneys," with the result that young wives "have illnesses that are difficult to treat" and "those who do not fall ill are also ruined."[6] Chu Cheng 褚澄, a doctor of the Southern Qi

[5] For a discussion of acupuncture and drug treatments for birth control and abortion in early imperial China, see Li Zhende, "Han Sui zhijian de 'shengzi buju' wenti," section entitled "Avoiding pregnancy, preventing birth, and inducing abortion," 787-94. Li Yinhe 李銀河 has researched the culture of birth in modern China and found that among women currently seventy to eighty years old, some had given birth seven, eight, or up to ten times. And among fifty- to sixty-year-old women who were not exposed to government family-planning policies, even without counting miscarriages and premature deaths, it was common to have five children. See Li Yinhe, *Shengyu yu zhongguo cunluo wenhua* 生育與中國村落文化 (Hong Kong: Oxford University Press, 1993), 109. Ebrey estimates that the average birth rate for a woman in the Song dynasty was about 6.1 children, and pregnancies that did not result in successful labor were even more numerous. See Ebrey, *Inner Quarters*, 172. When analyzing references to women and children in funeral inscriptions, I discovered that the average birth rate for an elite woman in the early imperial period was five children. One has to bear in mind, however, that the number of children a woman might have bore could have in reality been greater than this. Besides the fact that women died and were widowed earlier, some funeral texts mention only sons, but not daughters. For statistics on the age at which women died and were widowed, see Jen-der Lee, "The Life of Women in the Six Dynasties." Some scholars have suggested that the length of breastfeeding also assisted contraception. See Ping-chen Hsiung, "To Nurse the Young: Breastfeeding and Infant Feeding in Late Imperial China," *Journal of Family History* 20.3 (1995): 217-38. Regardless, quite a few women in early imperial China gave birth to approximately ten children according to extant historical materials. For the common people, if there was no concubine to share reproductive responsibilities with the main wife, a woman frequently might face death in pregnancy and at delivery.

[6] Chen Yanzhi's *Xiaopinfang* 小品方, cited in Tana Yasuyori 丹波康頼 (912-95), *Ishinpo* 醫心方 (982; Taipei: Xinwenfeng chubanshe; reprint of the Ansei woodblock edition, 1854), 21. 2a. Ma Jixing 馬繼興, in his "*Yixinfang* zhong de guyixue wenxian chutan" 醫心方中的古醫學文獻初探, *Nihon ishigaku zasshi* 日本醫史學雜誌 31.1 (1985): 326-71, estimates the period of composition for the *Xiaopinfang* to be the Jin dynasty (265-420). But after a fragmentary edition of the text was discovered in Japan in 1984,

(479-502), pointed out even more specifically that "frequent childbirth and nursing leads to blood withering and kills people."[7] He encouraged women to marry later and have fewer births, and proposed that "although, in men, essence penetrates at sixteen, they must not take a wife before thirty, and although women's reproductive capacities are developed at fourteen, they must not marry before twenty," otherwise "there will be intercourse, but no pregnancy, or pregnancy, but no birth, or birth, but the child will be fragile and not long-lived."[8]

In fact, there is no shortage of historical records of death due to childbirth. The Han dynasty (206 BCE- 220 CE) history recorded a shrine to *Shenjun* 神君, which was established because "a girl from Changling 長陵 died in childbirth and appeared as a spirit to her sister Wanruo 宛若. Wanruo set up a shrine for her in her room, and people came in masses to worship her."[9] The Jin 晉 dynasty (265-420) history recorded that Zhu Xianyi 諸顯夷, the wife of a certain Mi Yuanzong 米元宗, died at her home in childbirth.[10] Liu Yu 劉裕 (r. 420-22), the founding emperor of the Liu-Song dynasty, lost his mother on the day of his birth, and Yu was almost abandoned because of this.[11] The Liu-Song dynasty history also recorded that a certain Empress Zhao 趙 "died in the imperial Dantu 丹徒 palace due to childbirth complications, at the age of twenty-one."[12] The Chen dynasty (557-89) history recounted that Lady Sun 孫, the mother of King Wuxing called Yin 吳興王胤, "died in childbirth," and Yin was therefore raised by Empress Shen 沈.[13] There were nu-

---

some scholars consider that the author lived in the Liu-Song period. See Ren Xu 任旭, "*Xiaopinfang* canjuan jianjie" 小品方殘卷簡介, *Zhonghua yishi zazhi* 中華醫史雜誌 17.2 (1987): 71-73; and Liao Yuqun 廖育群, "Chen Yanzhi yu '*Xiaopinfang*' yanjiu de xin jinzhan" 陳延之與小品方研究的新進展, *Zhonghua yishi zazhi* 17.2 (1987): 74-75.

[7] Chu Cheng, *Chu Shi Yishu* 褚氏遺書 (Xinxiang: Henan kexue jishu chubanshe, 1986), "Jing xue" 精血, 33; "Wen zi" 問子, 57.

[8] Chu Cheng, *Chu Shi Yishu*, "Jing xue," 33; "Wen zi," 57.

[9] See Ban Gu 班固 (32-92), *Hanshu* 漢書 (Beijing: Zhonghua shuju, 1962), 25a.1216.

[10] Ganbao 干寶 (?-336), *Soushenji* 搜神記, cited in Li Fang 李昉 (925-96) ed, *Taiping guangji* 太平廣記 (Beijing: Renmin wenxue chubanshe, 1959, annotated ed.), 276.2186.

[11] Shen Yue 沈約 (441-513), *Songshu* 宋書 (Beijing: Zhonghua shuju, 1974), 47.1404.

[12] *Songshu*, 41.1280.

[13] Yao Silian 姚思廉 (557-637), *Chenshu* 陳書 (Beijing: Zhonghua shuju, 1972), 28.376.

merous examples of this kind.[14] Women of ancient times must have been quite conscious of the dangers of childbirth. The wife of the famous Han dynasty official Huo Guang 霍光 expressed this clearly: "In women's central affair of childbirth, ten die and one survives."[15] Chen Yanzhi described the time of women's delivery in the following way: "Getting down on the ground and squatting on straw [that is, delivery], in general is just like awaiting death."[16] One can see that the dangers of childbirth were certainly common knowledge among people of that time. The exploration of the process and meaning of childbirth therefore becomes an important angle for understanding the history of women's lives.

Childbirth might mean a woman's life or death, but its influence certainly was not limited to the mother's physical body. With regard to delivery, how did people in early imperial China respond? How was the progress of labor perceived by contemporary people? At what time was the birth completed? How did medical treatment and ritual behavior affect each other, and how were they interpreted in society? These issues are of great importance for understanding women's lives. Therefore, this article will use medical literature first to reconstruct the situation of women in the early imperial period in such practices as ensuring smooth delivery by taking herbal medicines during the last month of pregnancy, setting up a tent or arranging a hut for childbirth, squatting on straw as delivery time approached, management of obstetrical complications, and postpartum arrangements.[17] Then I will consult official histories, essays, and

---

[14] Childbirth related death also appeared in women's epitaphs of this period. For instance, Xue Huiming 薛慧命 of the Northern Wei (386-534) died of postpartum disorders when she lost her infant. See Zhao Wanli 趙萬里, *Han Wei Nanbeichao muzhi jishi*漢魏南北朝墓誌集釋 (Beijing: Kexue chubanshe, 1956), 4.32b.

[15] *Hanshu*, 97a.3966.

[16] *Xiaopinfang*, cited in *Ishinpo*, 23.25a.

[17] Medical records pre-dating the Tang have for the most part been lost. Fortunately, fragments are found in archaeological material and medical encyclopedia. The information used as evidence in this article relies mostly on Tana Yasuyori's *Ishinpo*, Sun Simiao's 孫思邈 (581-682) *Beiji qianjin yaofang* 備急千金要方 (Taipei: Hongye shuju reprint of Edo copy of Song dynasty woodblock edition, hereafter cited as *Qianjingfang*), and Wang Tao's 王燾 (ca. 670-755) *Waitai miyao* 外台秘要 (reprint of the Song edition, Taipei: Guoli zhongguo yiyao yanjiuso, 1964). In determining the date for each medical text, I have, for the most part, followed Nagasawa Motoho 長澤元夫 and Gotō Sirō 後藤志朗, "Inyōsyo kaisetsu" 引用書解說, in Ota Tenrei 太田典禮, *Ishinpo kaisetsu* (Tokyo: Nihon Koigaku siryō sennta-, 1973); and Ma Jixing, "Yixinfang zhong de guyixue wenxian chutan."

other materials in order to investigate the sociocultural implications of childbirth-related behavior.

Several points should be made before we proceed further. First, although the time period of this article is defined as early imperial China, in some cases, I use source material from periods before the Han and after the Tang dynasty (618-906). Owing to the continuity of the social history and the medical tradition, it is impossible in this research to differentiate developments strictly by dynastic periodization.[18] Second, because of the vastness of China's territory and potential variations in local customs, regional distinctions should certainly be considered. But in view of the difficulties in gathering material related to the culture of childbirth, unless historical sources specifically point to the special characteristics of a region, this article will first consider the ideas shared by the people of that time and leave local diversities to further research.[19]

In addition to the influence of time and space, childbearing women and their families might have reacted differently in childbirth according to differing social status. The received medical literature was, after all, written by literate people and was generally directed

[18] First of all, we see similar concepts and continuous knowledge regarding fetal development in the *Taichanshu* 胎產書, unearthed from the Han dynasty tomb at Mawangdui; Xu Zhicai's 徐之才 *Zhuyue yangtaifang* 逐月養胎方 from the Northern Qi (550-577); and the *Chanjing* 產經 of the Sui dynasty. Second, although texts like the *Luyanfang* 錄驗方 and *Qianjinfang* were probably completed in the early Tang, their writers, Zhen Quan 甄權 (540-643) and Sun Simiao had indeed lived through the three dynasties of the Northern Zhou, Sui, and Tang. The records in the texts therefore responded to gynecological and obstetrical expositions and prescriptions from the Six Dynasties on. Lastly, *Waitai miyao* by the mid-Tang writer Wang Tao contains records from many lost medical texts from the Six Dynasties and early Tang. For information on the relationship between the Mawangdui *Taichanshu* and later ideas on nurturing the fetus, see Ma Jixing, *Taichanshu* kaoshi 胎產書考釋, in *Mawangdui guyishu kaoshi* 馬王堆古醫書考釋 (Changsha: Hunan kexue jishu chubanshe, 1992); Li Jianmin, "Mawangdui hanmu boshu 'Yuzang maibaotu' jianzheng", 754-55, appendix. Both the *Chanjing* and the "Zhujue yangtaifang" are lost and part of the contents of the former is included in *Ishinpo*, while the latter included in *Qianjingfang*. As for the *Luyanfang*, Liu Xu 劉昫 (887-946), *Jiu Tangshu* 舊唐書, "Jingjizhi"經籍志 (Beijing: Zhonghua shuju, 1975), 47.2050, recorded an "ancient *Luyanfang* in 50 scrolls, composed by Zhen Quan." And as for Zhen Quan, in the *Jiu Tangshu*, "Fangji zhuan" 方技傳, 191.1089-90, recorded that he lived through the Northern Zhou, Sui, and early Tang periods and died at the age of 103 (540-643).

[19] Cultivating medicinal plants seems to have become increasingly widespread, causing a reduction of regional differences. Generally speaking, the herbs used in prescriptions of contemporary medical literature seemed to have mostly come from Sichuan, the Northwest, and the North of China. See the discussion below.

at the upper classes. However, from extant medical literature, it is difficult to know whether the refinement or vulgarity in how both official families and ordinary groups dealt with childbirth was determined by the availability of resources or devergent concepts.[20] From reading these texts, we can at least know that by the seventh century, between the Sui (581-618) and the Tang (618-907) dynasties, doctors seem to have become increasingly dissatisfied with the concepts and methods of childbirth of their time and to have aimed for improvement. In the end, what images of childbirth can we see in the the medical texts? And how was this related to society's customs and the situation of women? This article will discuss these issues in the following three sections: "Entering the Month," "Delivery," and "Postpartum."

Entering the Month

Medical texts after the Song dynasty often called the beginning of the last month of pregnancy "entering the month" and advised treating the pregnant woman with special care.[21] Among the medical

[20] For example, the practice of burying the placenta after birth in order to ensure the child's longevity could have been a popular concept, but the common people might not necessarily have buried placentas according to the complex procedure prescribed in the chart excavated from Mawangdui. Divining the newborn's fate might also have been a popular idea, but it might not have always followed the description of "Neize" 內則, *Liji* 禮記, *Shisanjing zhushuben* 十三經注疏本 (Taipei: Yiwen yinshuguan, 1955) where "the fortuneteller carried out the task within three days." As for delivery itself, while there might have been regional or class differences in the herbs and implements to assist in the birth, the medicines, implements, and taboos and restrictions all clearly suggest shared notions that "a speedy and painless birth constituted a smooth delivery" and that "all things resonate with each other." See detailed discussion below. With regard to placenta burial customs, see Li Jianmin, "Mawangdui Hanmu boshu 'Yuzang maibaotu' jianzheng"; for divining the newborn's fate, see Poo Mu-chou 蒲慕州, "Shuihudi Qinjian rishu de shijie" 睡虎地秦簡日書的世界, in *Bulletin of the Institute of History and Philology, Academia Sinica* 62.4 (1993): 623-75; Anne Behnke Kinney, "Infant Abandonment in Early China," *Early China* 18 (1993): 107-38.

[21] Wang Huai-yin 王懷隱 (ca. 925-97) ed., *Taiping Shenghuifang* 太平聖惠方 (reprint of the Song woodblock edition; Osaka: Oriento shubānsha, 1991), 76.20-21, stated that the medicines given in preparation for childbirth should "all be sufficiently ready on the first day of entering the month," "the delivering woman may not drink wine after entering the month," and "in front of a house where a woman is entering the month, no one may stop, leavc traces, or stay overnight," etc. Chen Ziming's 陳自明 (ca. 1190-1270) *Furen daquan liangfang* 婦人大全良方(Beijing: Renmin weisheng

prescriptions for assisting childbirth pre-dating the Tang, the term "entering the month" also occurred, but the complete set of systems and rules to protect this stage of pregnancy seems not to have been clearly defined yet, and it was only the aspects of taking medicines to make the fetus slippery and setting up a tent and arranging a hut that were specified.

a) *Taking Medicines to Make the Fetus Slippery*

Medicinal decoctions to promote a smooth birth seem to have increased gradually in complexity. In a few instances explanations for taking medicines differ from one medical text to another in the early period, but they were later standardized. The *Taichanshu* 胎產書 (Book for childbirth), that was unearthed from the Han tomb at Mawangdui 馬王堆, contains the following record: "One who carries a child should boil the heads of *baimugou* 白牡狗 and eat them all by herself. Her child will be beautiful and dazzling, and it will emerge easily."[22] "*Mugou* heads" has been interpreted as *muloushou* 牡螻首 "mole cricket heads," that is, *lougu* 螻蛄, "mole crickets," a recipe popularly known in early China for treating retained placenta.[23] Other scholars suggest that the two terms "boil" and "eat all by herself" show that what is referred to is not a small insect like the mole cricket, but the head of a male dog of white color, which might be related to notions of dog blood curing childbirth complications

chubanshe, 1985) vol. 16, also includes a chapter on "medicines to be prepared for entering the month." Zhu Duanzhang 朱端章 (ca. twelfth century), *Weisheng jiabao chanke beiyao* 衛生家寶產科備要 (1184; Shanghai: Sanlian shuju, 1990) collected all kinds of obstetrical texts and specifically mentioned that when "entering the month" one should prepare all the medicines needed for delivery and postpartum care, select a midwife, arrange the birthing room, hang up the delivery chart, clearly understand the position of the directions for burying the placenta, and make the mother take a daily dose of birth-protecting pills; also, a rule prohibits the mother washing her hair. See Zhu Duanzhang, *Weisheng jiabao chanke beiyao*, 1.1; 1.3; 6.65. Ebrey also points out that Song obstetrical and gynecological books paid special attention to "entering the month"; see her *The Inner Quarters*, 173.

[22] Ma Jixing, *Mawangdui guyishu kaoshi*, 806.

[23] From the Han on, people believed that mole crickets had the effect of treating retained placenta. Cui Shi 崔寔 (103-70), *Simin yueling* 四民月令 (Beijing: Nongye chubanshe, 1981), stated that on the fifth day of the fifth month, "one can make mincemeat … with … east-moving mole crickets," and cites from the Northern Wei agricultural book *Qimin Yaoshu* 齊民要術, saying that "mole crickets have stings; remove the sting for treating childbirth complications and retained placenta."

and breech presentation and dog hair used in curing childbirth complications.[24]

The Han doctor Zhang Zhongjing 張仲景 (145-208) and the Jin doctor Wang Shuhe 王叔和 proposed that pregnant women should regularly take angelica powder. Grinding angelica, scutellaria, peony, ligusticum, and ovate atryctulodes into powder and taking it in liquor twice a day is said to "ease childbirth and cause the fetus to be healthy and without suffering when taken constantly in pregnancy. After birth it also controls the myriad illnesses." [25] Moreover, for heaviness of the body and inhibited urination in pregnancy, one should take mallow seed and poria powder, as Xu Zhongke (452-536) stated, "Mallow can make the fetus slippery."[26] Tao Hongjing 陶弘景 said, "Plant mallow in the fall, raise it through the winter, and when it produces seeds in the spring, it is called winter mallow. Added to medicine, its nature makes the medicine slippery and flowing."[27] Chen Yanzhi's *Xiaopinfang* 小品方 (Recipes of small pieces) stated that "fritillaria causes easy childbirth."[28] Nevertheless, none of the above-mentioned medical

[24] See Zhou Yimou 周一謀 and Xiao Zuotao 蕭佐桃, *Mawangdui yishu kaozhu* 馬王堆醫書考注 (Tianjin: Kexue jishu chubanshe, 1989), 355, quoting Tao Hongjing 陶弘景 (452-536) *Mingyi bielu* 名醫別錄, and Su Jing's 蘇敬 remarks from the Tang dynasty. Ma Jixing subsequently translates "eat alone" as "only eating mole crickets." If this is correct, then this would constitute a recipe to facilitate the final stage of delivery, see *Mawangdui guyishu kaoshi*, 806.

[25] Zhang Zhongjing (145-208), *Jingui yaolüe* 金匱要略, annotated by Xu Zhongke 徐忠可 (Beijing: Renmin weisheng chubanshe, 1993), 20.304. Wang Shuhe (ca. fourth c.), *Maijing* 脈經 (Sibu congkan chubian ed. 四部叢刊初編本; Shanghai: Shanghai shudian, 1965), 9.4b. Li Shizhen 李時珍 (1518-93), *Bencao gangmu* 本草綱目 (Beijing: Renmin weisheng chubanshe, 1975-81), "Herbs," 14.2-5, recorded that, "*Bielu* 別錄 states: 'Angelica grows in river valleys of west Gansu.' Su Song 蘇頌 stated: 'Now it is available in the various prefectures of Sichuan and Shaanxi, as well as Jiangning prefecture and Chuzhou, among which the one from Sichuan is the best.'" For English translation and Latin names of the herbs mentioned in this article, I rely mostly on Nigel Wiseman and Feng Ye, eds., *A Practical Dictionary of Chinese Medicine* (Brookline, Mass: Paradigm Publications, 1998).

[26] Zhang Zhongjing, *Jingui yaolüe*, 20.302-3.

[27] Zhan Yin's 昝殷 *Chan Bao* 產寶 from the Tang dynasty also recommended winter mallow to treat breech presentation. Li Shizhen also suggested that mallow could "relax the orifices, increase lactation, reduce swelling, and make the fetus slippery"; moreover, the roots and leaves could be used identically to the seed. In terms of its geographical origin, the *Bielu* states that "winter mallow seeds originate at Shaoshi mountain 少室山"; Su Song from the Song dynasty stated that "mallow is available everywhere." See *Bencao gangmu*, "Herbs," 16.88-91.

[28] *Xiaopinfang*, quoted in *Waitai miyao*, 33.291. It also said that "in the last month of pregnancy when one develops spasms due to Wind," or when depression and vomiting

texts specified at what time one should ingest medicinal decoctions to make the fetus slippery. It was said that angelica "when taken regularly in pregnancy will ease birth," and, like mallow, fritillaria, and similar herbs, it appeared regularly in the medical prescriptions for treating childbirth complications. In view of this, there might have been the risk of miscarriage if taken at the beginning of pregnancy, and it could therefore be used only at the end of pregnancy.[29]

Besides mole crickets, angelica, and mallow seeds, the medical text *Seng Shen fang* 僧深方 (Recipes of Master Shen) from the fifth century stated that salvia paste is able to nurture the fetus and ease birth. Salvia paste contained salvia, ginseng, angelica, ligusticum, Sichuan pepper, and ovate atryctulodes, decocted in pig lard and to be ingested with heated wine. The *Seng Shen fang* stated that "one can take it from the seventh month of pregnancy on. It will cause one to give birth all of a sudden, lying or sitting, without sensation, and it also treats postpartum stasis pain."[30] The *Chanjing* 產經 (Birth canon), of the sixth century, claimed that "in the seventh month of pregnancy, one may regularly take salvia paste, so that, sitting or lying, one may give birth without sensation."[31] However, Xu Zhicai 徐之才 (492-572) suggested that it can only be taken in the tenth month of pregnancy, thus revealing discrepancies in opinions of contemporary

occur, one can add fritillaria to the decoction. The *Luyanfang* said that "when made into a powder and taken with wine, fritillaria can treat complications in childbirth and a retained placenta." Quoted in Tang Wanchun 湯萬春, *Xiaopinfang jilu jianzhu* 小品方輯錄箋注 (Hefei: Anhui kexue jishu chubanshe, 1990), 21.109-10.

[29] Zhu Duanzhang, *Weisheng jiabao chanke beiyao*, 6.65, quoted in *Yushi beichan jiyong fang* 虞氏備產濟用方: "After the first five months of pregnancy, it is suitable to take 'trifoliate orange decoction' to make the fetus slippery." The same text, 6.73, also said: "This recipe is miraculous; it will cause a slippery fetus and easy birth, other medicines cannot measure up to it.... For a birthing woman who is usually depleted and weak, one should exercise greater caution because trifoliate orange is cold in nature and she should probably not take too much of it." *Weisheng jiabao chanke beiyao*, 7.95: "Trifoliate orange powder, taken from the fifth month of pregnancy on, can normalize *qi*, thin the fetus, and ease birth." The same text, 7.96, also introduced another delivery-easing recipe that should be taken regularly only from the fifth or sixth month on. From this we get the impression that these medicinal decoctions for slippery fetus should at the very least only be taken after the fifth or sixth month of pregnancy.

[30] *Sengshenfang* cited in *Ishinpo*, 22.18ab. *Sengshenfang* is recorded in Wei Zheng 魏徵 (580-643), *Zhangsun Wuji* 長孫無忌 (?-659) ed., *Suishu* 隋書 "Jingjizhi" 經籍志 (Beijing: Zhonghua shuju, 1973), 34.1042 as authored by Shisengshen 釋僧深 (ca. sixth c.).

[31] *Chanjing* quoted in *Ishinpo*, 23.9a; 22.18b. According to Nagasawa and Gotō, the *Chanjing* was authored by De Zhenchang 德貞常 of the Sui dynasty.

doctors.[32] In medical recipes for assisting birth in the tenth-century *Taiping shenghuifang* 太平聖惠方 (Recipes of imperial grace from the Taiping era), it was said that "salvia paste should be given at the time of pregnancy in advance in order to move the fetus forward and make it slippery." In the twelfth century, Zhu Duanzhang's 朱端章 *Weisheng jiabao chanke beiyao* 衛生家寶產科備要 (Precious family guide to protecting life in childbirth; ca. 1184) specifically adopts Xu Zhicai's view of taking it only when entering the last month, and the suggestion of taking it in the seventh month does not reappear.[33]

In addition to salvia paste, women in the final stage of pregnancy could also take "licorice powder," made from a combination of licorice, scutellaria, dried bean sprouts, nonglutinous rice, sesame seed, dried ginger, cinnamon bark, and evodia. The *Xiaopinfang* suggested that one should start taking it "one month before the day of birth and, after thirty days, one will be able to move around as usual and does not even notice it when the child is born and dropped to the ground."[34] The *Qianjinfang* 千金方 (Recipes worth a thousand gold pieces) recorded a birth-easing medicine made from a combination of plantago seeds, ass-hide glue, and talcum. It strongly advised taking it "only in the month of birth. The medicine 'relaxes the nine orifices', and one should not take it earlier."[35] These two are thus medicinal prescriptions for making the fetus slippery and assisting in birth that can be taken only in the month of birth.

Elite families were able to increase protection and care for a pregnant woman in the final stage, as recommended in the medical texts. The common people might also have had ideas regarding herbal medicines to make the fetus slippery, but even if they did, we do not know whether they were able to take medicine according to the recipes.

b) *Setting up a Tent and Arranging a Hut*

In addition to promoting smooth labor with medicinal prescriptions for a slippery fetus during the last months of pregnancy, elite house-

---

32 Xu Zhicai, *Zhuyue yangtaifang* 逐月養胎方, cited in Sun Simiao, *Qianjinfang*, 2.24.

33 Zhu Duanzhang, *Weisheng jiabao chanke beiyao*, 2.24.

34 *Xiaopingfang* cited in *Waitai miyao*, 34.941. As for the geographical origin of licorice, the *Bencao ganmu* stated that "it first grows in the valleys west of the Yellow river; later it comes from Sichuan and, in the Song, [and it] is available in all prefectures of Shaanxi and Hedong." See *Bencao gangmu*, "Herbs," 12.81-85.

35 *Qianjinfang*, 2.25.

holds were also more likely to prepare in advance a location for the pregnant woman to deliver. Choosing and preparing a location for the expectant mother was an important task by the last month of pregnancy. The *Chanjing* is the earliest extant medical text to mention preparing a birth quarter for the pregnant woman. The birth quarter might have been specially constructed outside or set up a room inside the house. A birth quarter erected outside was called a "birth hut," *chanlu* 產廬. The *Chanjing* stated that "it is auspicious to position the birth hut according to the direction of the month," and, "Whenever making a birth hut... it is forbidden to place it on fresh-cut wheat stalks or under tall trees, great misfortune! Do not place it near the stove sacrifice—also great misfortune!"[36] Thus, it is quite possible that the birth hut was a slight distance away from the residence.

An outdoor birth quarter was also sometimes referred to as a "birth tent," *chanzhang* 產帳, but "birth tent" did not necessarily always refer to a birth quarter outdoors. The *Waitai miyao* 外臺祕要 (Secret essentials from the Imperial Palace) proposed that, when searching for a location for delivery, "if the spirits are outside, give birth inside the house; if they are inside, give birth outside. Place the birth tent in an empty space of auspicious virtue. To determine a space of auspicious virtue inside the house, also rely on the tent-erecting method."[37] Thus, apparently, the term "birth tent" could refer to a birth quarter erected both indoors or outdoors. It was recorded that on the day after Empress Wucheng 武成 (r.561-564) of the Northern Qi gave birth, "there was an owl crying on top of the birth tent."[38] We can assume in this case that the birth tent was probably erected outdoors, and the term "tent" was not necessarily identical to the screen curtains that were set around the birthing woman's bed,

[36] *Chanjing*, quoted in *Ishinpo* 23.8a. *Chanjing* also states "in the first, sixth, seventh, and eleventh months of the year, make a hut with one entrance, always facing southeast for good luck. In the second, third, fourth, fifth, eighth, ninth, tenth, and twelfth months, make a birth hut with one entrance, always facing southwest for good luck." quoted in *Ishinpo*, 23.8ab.

[37] *Waitai miyao*, 33.927.

[38] Li Baiyao 李百藥 (565-648), *Bei Qi shu* 北齊書 (Beijing: Zhonghua shuju, 1972), 9.126. However, Li Fang 李昉 (925-96), *Taiping yulan* 太平御覽 (Taipei: Commercial Press, reprint of the Song edition, 1967), 701.7a, quoted Gan Bao, *Soushenji*, saying that, "There was a Miss Zhang in Changan who stayed alone in her house when a pigeon entered from outside and stopped on her bed." This shows that it did happen that wild birds flew into houses.

which was often the case after the Song dynasty.[39] Moreover, it did not refer to a screen curtain set around the ordinary sleeping bed, but was prepared specifically for the woman in labor:

> The *Sushuo* 俗說 said: When Huan Xuan 桓玄 was in Nanzhou, his concubine was about to give birth and was afraid of Wind and therefore needed a tent. Huan said, "There is no need to make a tent. She can use my main wife's old tent."[40]

This example shows that the birth tent was a structure made in advance for the laboring woman, maybe with the goal of avoiding wind. But from the care doctors put into setting up the tent, we can see that their considerations were not limited to merely avoiding wind.

The method for erecting the tent relied on birth charts. The *Chanjing* and the *Waitai miyao* guided the expectant mother's household in how to set up a hut or tent in accordance with the divinatory direction of the month. This particular attention paid to time and direction in accordance with the birth charts was already practiced in early China. The various types of birth charts seem to have undergone development between the Han and Tang in which the content gradually became consistent and the principles standardized. Evidence in the *Taichanshu* reflects that there used to be a separate chart for burying the placenta. According to earlier research, the delivery room was to be taken as the center from which an auspicious place was chosen among twelve positions in an outside square of the four cardinal directions.[41]

The *yiwenzhi* 藝文志 (bibliography section) in the *Suishu* recorded two scrolls of "birth charts" *chantu* 產圖 and four scrolls of "various birth charts" *zachantu* 雜產圖, but their exact content is unclear.[42] As for the position of the woman giving birth, before the sixth century *Chanjing*, there were already instructional manuals and charts to

---

[39] The phrase *chanzhang* after the Song often referred to a screened curtain set up around the pregnant woman's bed. *Taiping shenghui fang*, 76.31b, said that "when entering the first day of the birth month, write a copy of the birth chart, [and] stick it directly in the birth tent on the north-facing wall." *Weisheng jiabao chanke beiyao*, 1.1, says "for all births, on the first day of entering the month, stick a birth chart on the north-facing wall inside the bedroom."

[40] *Taiping yulan*, 699.4b.

[41] See Ma Jixing, *Mawangdui guyishu kaoshi*, 764; Li Jianmin, "Mawangdui Hanmu boshu 'Yuzang maibao tu' jianzheng."

[42] *Suishu*, 34.1037.

help the family determine the direction in which the laboring woman should squat. However, according to De Zhenchang 德貞常, the author of the *Chanjing*, most of these manuals had too many and confusing instructions and were difficult to understand. De Zhenchang wrote a revised manual for choosing the sitting direction called the "Twelve Month Charts" *shieryuetu* 十二月圖. The *Chanjing* stated that "it is clear and easy to understand. Whenever there is a birth, one should always rely on this without ever again using the other spirit charts."[43] Obviously De Zhenchang made an effort to integrate various earlier charts and strove hard for consistency. The *Chanjing* quoted in the *Ishinpo* 醫心方 (Recipes of the heart of medicine), does not contain an actual copy of the Month Charts, *yuetu* 月圖, but according to *Chanjing*'s annotations to these charts recorded in *Ishinpo*, their most important function was to match the three factors of the month of childbirth, the direction, and the posture in which to await birth, in order to avoid the presence of various spirits and to find an auspicious place for delivery. For example, "in the first month, the Heavenly *Qi* 氣 flows south, the woman in labor should face south and kneel with her left knee touching the earth in the *bing* 丙 location; this is great fortune," and so on.[44]

Since the *Chanjing* was lost and the Month Charts were not included in the *Ishinpo*, it is impossible to know whether the "Twelve Month Charts" of the *Chanjing* recorded only the direction and position of the woman in labor, or whether it also specified the auspicious locations for setting up the tent and burying the placenta. If it indeed only marked the position for squatting, then it was an independent birth chart of a separate category, similar to the *Yuzang maibao tu* 禹藏埋胞圖 (Placenta-burial chart of Yu) found in the Mawangdui *Taichanshu*. However, a comparison of the annotations in the sixth-century *Chanjing* with the birth charts recorded in the eighth-century *Waitai miyao*, the tenth-century *Taiping Shenghuifang*, and the twelfth-century *Weisheng jiabao chanke beiyao* proves two facts. First, the

---

[43] *Ishinpo* 23.2b.

[44] *Ishinpo* 23.3a-5b offers examples for the postures and directions which the laboring woman should face from the first to the twelfth month. For detailed discussion on the selection of Chinese texts and figures by Tana Yasuyori in his *Ishinpo* and its significance to Chinese and Japanese gynecological and obstetric medicine, see Li Zhende (Jen-der Lee), "*Ishinpo* lun furen zhubing soyou jiqi xiangguan wenti" 醫心方論婦人諸病所由及其相關問題, *Tsing Hua Journal of Chinese Studies* 清華學報 34.2 (2004): 495-511.

Chanjing basically belonged to the same system as the three charts from the later periods, and the direction considered auspicious in each month is for the most part identical.[45] Second, the three charts from later periods combined setting up the tent, arranging birth, and burying the placenta--functions that had individual charts earlier--into one chart (see Figures 1 and 2).

The *Taiping Shenghuifang* pointed out, "For positioning the laboring woman and burying the placenta, in both cases, a location should be arranged inside (the house) to pick an auspicious place. For burying the placenta and various filths, this should be a place indoors. Whenever determining the place for the laboring woman, this is the location of the *yuekong* 月空 (monthly emptiness); one should do it accordingly. Make a hole ahead of time and, when everything is finished, cover it back up."[46] The *Weisheng jiabao chanke beiyao* further clarified that "all places for arranging the birth and burying the placenta should be distributed inside the bedroom."[47] This shows that, at the latest from the eighth century on, there were already charts that incorporated the various tasks of delivery into one standardized birth chart, and that, at the latest from the tenth century on, the birth chart was hung inside the birthing room so that arranging the birth and burying the placenta were all carried out according to the chart.

It is clear from the above discussion that doctors thought that, under ideal circumstances in terms of time, finances, and labor, a family with an impending birth should search out and arrange a location for delivery according either to separate or synthesized charts after the mother entered the last month of pregnancy. However, the time of delivery was up to Heaven, not to people, and there was no way to propel the action. If the month passed without the woman's giving birth, the medical texts suggested that everything be changed according to the next month's chart.[48] But sometimes delivery hap-

---

[45] But one needs to be aware that, while they basically follow the same system, the auspicious location mentioned in the *Waitai miyao* for setting up the laboring woman's tent is in the *Chanjing* the place where she should squat, and the two charts after the tenth century called the auspicious location a place for "arranging delivery," *anchan* 安產, instead of "setting up the tent for the laboring woman," *anchanfuzhang* 安產婦帳. Whether in the end the birth tent was placed inside the house around the bed or on the ground might also have been uncertain.

[46] *Taiping shenghuifang*, 76.32.

[47] *Weisheng jiabao chanke beiyao*, 1.1.

[48] *Weisheng jiabao chanke beiyao*, 1.1.

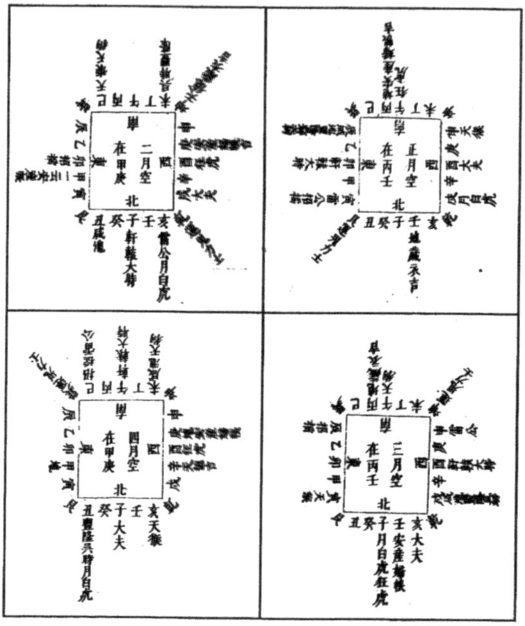

Figure 1: Birth chart (for the first four months) from the seventh-century *Cuishi*, recorded in the eighth-century *Waitai miyao*.

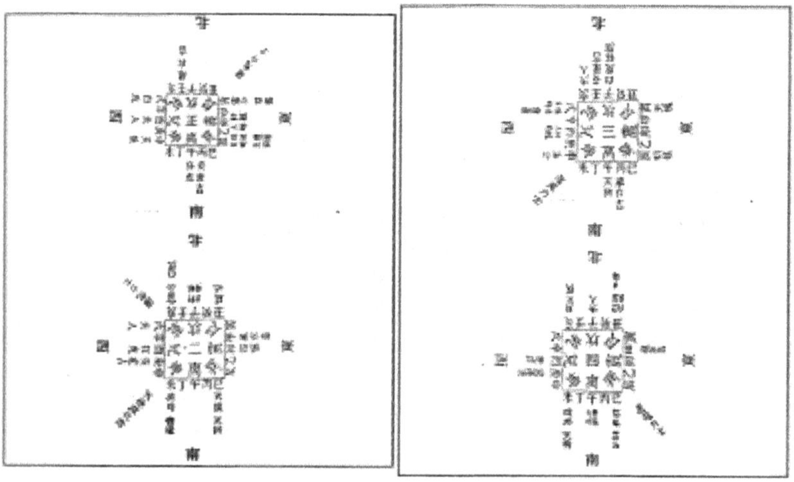

Figure 2: Birth chart (for the first four months) recorded in twelfth-century *Weisheng jiabao chanke beiyao*.

pened suddenly, not allowing people time to prepare. What instructions did medical texts offer once the labor pains started? The three sections below on 'Sitting on straw,' 'Assisting in birth' and 'Saving complications' discuss women's childbirth procedures in this early imperial period.

Delivery

People approached delivery with great worry and fear, and elite households would have made many preparations after entering the month. But once labor started, they had to manage the situation on the spot. With respect to determining when this important time would arrive, the *yiwenzhi* in the *Suishu* recorded one volume by Wang Chen 王琛 (ca. sixth century) titled 'Method for predicting when a pregnant woman will give birth,' and one volume called 'Method for predicting birth'. It was said that a sixth-century doctor Xu Zun 許遵 instructed his son Xu Hui 許暉 in a "method for predicting women's labors, foretelling the sex of the newborns and the days of birth, and he never missed it."[49] But given the fact that Xu Hui was "rewarded several times for this [his calculations]"[50] in Emperor Wucheng's 武成 reign (r.561-564), it is obvious that to predict the time of birth was an extraordinary skill not within the reach of ordinary people. Xu Zhicai's *Zhuyue yangtaifang* (Recipes to nourish the fetus each month) and the section on pregnancy in Sun Simiao's *Qianjinfang* merely stated, "When the days are full, then she will give birth,"[51] and "Wait for the time and give birth." This shows that predicting the time of birth was difficult, and, for the most part, people just had to be patient and wait. But how were things handled once labor started? The annotations to the chart in the *Chanjing* quoted above not only pointed out the suitable and the forbidden directions, but also told women in labor to await birth touching the ground with one knee. Thus women were apparently not lying in bed when approaching delivery but taking a vertical position, such as kneeling and touching the ground. I will first discuss the posture of women giving birth.

---

[49] *Suishu*, 34.1037.

[50] Li Yanshou 李延壽 (ca. seventh century), *Beishi* 北史 (Beijing: Zhonghua shuju, 1974), 89.2936.

[51] *Qianjinfang*, 2.24.

a) *Getting on the Ground and Sitting on Straw*

Information regarding "getting on the ground and sitting on straw," which indicates a vertical position for delivery, emerged since the pre-imperial period. Scholars believe that one of the female carved stone figures unearthed from the archaeological site of Houtaizu 后台子 in Hebei reflects a posture of squatting during delivery.[52] In terms of information from the medical literature, the section on 'infant-cord rigidity' (*yinger suojing* 嬰兒索痙) in the Mawangdui *Wushier bingfang* 五十二病方 (Recipes for fifty-two diseases) stated: "As for cord rigidity, if at the time of birth [she] remains on moist ground for too long, the flesh becomes stiff and the mouth clenched, the sinews curled up and difficult to stretch out." Although scholars disagree on who the patient suffering from the condition of infant cord rigidity is, some saying the birthing mother, some saying the infant, nevertheless, the explanation of "remaining" as "sitting" proves that delivery occurred mostly by sitting on the ground since ancient China.[53]

The fifth-century doctor Chen Yanzhi said, "In ancient times, women gave birth by getting on the ground and sitting on straw, just like awaiting death."[54] On the one hand, this reflects the dangers of childbirth, and on the other it seems to indicate that in ancient times delivery mostly occurred in a sitting position.[55] Since

---

[52] For the report and pictures of the figure, see Chengde diqu wenwubaoguansuo 承德地區文物保管所, Luanpingxian bowuguan 灤平縣博物館, "Hebei Luanpingxian houtaizi yizhi fajue jianbao" 河北灤平縣后台子遺址發掘簡報, *Wenwu* 文物 3 (1994): 53-74. For the meaning of the stone figurines, see Tang Chi湯池, "Shilun Luanping houtaizi chutu de shidiao nüshenxiang" 試論灤平后台子出土的石雕女神像, *Wenwu* 3 (1994): 46-51.

[53] Ma Jixing thought that the woman developed tetany from sitting on wet ground too long during childbirth. See his *Mawangdui guyishu kaoshi*, 368-69. Zhou Yimou thinks that this entry was to describe the newborn instead of the mother. See Zhou Yimou and Xiao Zuotao, *Mawangdui yishu kaozhu*, 71-72. For English translation and interpretation of this disorder, see Donald Harper, *Early Chinese Medical Literature: the Mawangdui Medical Manuscripts* (London: Kegan Paul, 1998), 231-32.

[54] Quoted from *Ishinpo*, 23.25a.

[55] Ancient people sat on the ground in different positions. Scholars suggest that there were at least two positions, kneeling *gui* 跪 and sitting *zuo* 坐. The former is to stand on one's knees so that the body from the knees upward forms a straight line. The latter is to sit on one's heels so that the body from the buttocks upward forms a straight line. In addition, there was squatting and sitting with the legs sprawled out, both considered rude in ancient China. See Li Ji 李濟, "Gui, zuo, dunju yu jiju" 跪坐蹲居與箕踞, *Bulletin of the Institute of History and Philology, Academia Sinica,* 24 (1953):

this is called the method of birth in "ancient times," did a different method of giving birth appear in the Six Dynasties? Touching the ground with one knee, as mentioned in the *Chanjing*, seems to refer to giving birth kneeling. Chao Yuanfang's 巢元方(ca. sixth-seventh c.) *Zhubing yuanhoulun* 諸病源候論 (Essays on the origins and signs of diseases; referred to below as *Bingyuanlun* 病源論) says that:

> Women give birth either sitting or lying. If she gives birth sitting, she should sit erect and the attendants should support her by holding her around the waist. They should not allow her to bend over so that the child can follow its natural course without hindrance. As for giving birth lying down, she should also lie steadily, her back should be level and touch the mat, her body not bent or crooked so the child will not lose its way."[56]

From the perspective of modern obstetrical knowledge, in supine deliveries, the mother is immobolized on her back, and the uterus presses aginst the vena cava, causing both the mother and the baby to suffer.[57] Moreover, at the stage when she thinks of pushing out the child due to abdominal pain, she might be more inclined to squat rather than lie down, therefore giving birth in the supine position seems rather unnatural in terms of basic physiology. In view of this, the statements in *Bingyuanlun* seem better understood as advice for different situations instead of requirements for delivery. What it means is that if the woman was sitting, she should sit straight and not bend over, and if she was lying, then her back should be level and touching the mat, not bent and crooked. In *Waitai miyao* a case was described in which the woman in labor was advised by the doctor to "sit or to lie down at will," but still mainly exerted her strength when squatting.

> The woman's abdomen hurt, which seemed to be the symptom of birth. I then told [her family] to move away the beds and tables, spread grass in three or four places on the ground, hang down ropes and tie them to wood to make a horizontal bar, measure the height to her armpits when squatting, to allow her to lean against it like a crossbeam. Below I spread out blankets, for fear that the child might drop on the straw and injure itself. When the preparations were completed in this manner, I let the person in labor assume her position, telling her to sit or lie down at will, explaining the method [of delivery] to her.[58]

283-301. Although a woman in labor might have touched the ground with her knee, it seems that the position of squatting was most frequent. See discussion below.

[56] *Bingyuanlun*, 43.4.

[57] Michel Odent, *Birth Reborn* (Medford, N.J.: Birth Works Press, 1984), 96.

[58] *Waitai miyao*, 33.924. Here Wang Tao was actually citing from *Cuishi* 崔氏, most

In reality, the legs might have grown numb in a squatting position, and this position could not be sustained for too long. Thus, the woman in labor might have chosen whatever posture she felt comfortable in or was used to, sometimes squatting, sometimes standing up, changing positions in order to exert her strength best. Still, squatting was most common, and therefore she needed something to lean on.[59] The laboring woman in the *Waitai miyao* leaned on a crossbar; the mother in Yang Zijian's 楊子建 (ca. eleventh century.) *Shichanlun* 十產論 (Essays on ten birth methods) dating from the Northern Song dynasty held on to a cloth:

> The tenth [way of delivery] is called giving birth in a sitting position. A sitting birth means that when the child is about to be born, one should firmly suspend a hand cloth from a high place, and make the laboring woman grasp it with her hands. She should crouch down ever so slightly into a sitting position to allow the child to be born, but she may not sit down and block the path of child's birth.[60]

Sometimes she might have held on to or leaned on other things due to prohibition of certain objects on the day of birth. On certain days, the *Waitai miyao* says, "she cannot hold on to a rope, but instead a horse's bit should be suspended for her to hold; this is auspicious."[61] Thus it appears that ordinarily a crossbar might not have been made, but the women held directly onto a rope. Otherwise, there would be people who held her waist from behind to assist in labor; as described in *Bingyuanlun*, "attendants should support her by holding her around the waist." The *Waitai miyao* also said, "Again, in all methods for delivery, one must wait patiently, and must not rush it by force. Wait until the child hurts and wants to come out and only afterwards hold her waist. The attendants must not be startled or alarmed or handle things in a dissolute manner."[62] A horse's bit was not an item ordinarily available to the common people on small farms, but was mostly used by elite households. In order to suspend rope and tie wood to it, there must have been

---

likely written by Cui Zhiti 崔知悌 (d. 681), whose works on childbirth medicine were also included in the dynastic histories of the Tang. Textual analysis and discussion on Cui's work and Wang's citation, see Jen-der Lee, "Gender and Medicine in Tang China" *Asia Major* 16.2 (2003): 1-32.

59 Doctors also point out that it helps the woman to relax if she changes positions in labor. See Odent, *Birth Reborn*, 98.

60 Chen Ziming, *Furen daquan liangfang*, 463-68, quoting Yang Zijian.

61 *Waitai miyao*, 33.927, quoting "Cuishi nianli chengtufa" 崔氏年立成圖法.

62 *Waitai miyao*, 33.924.

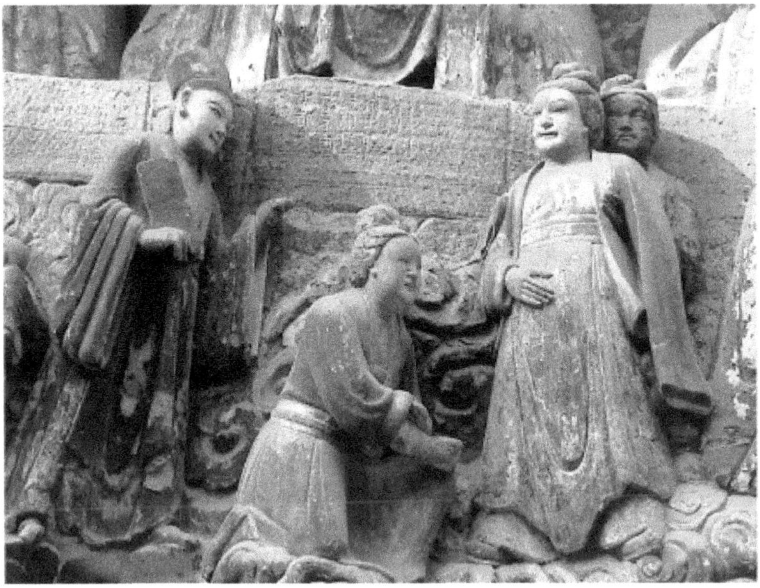

Figure 3: Scene of delivery in the *Fumu enzhongjing* sculpture, Dazu, Sichuan (Photograph by the author).

enough space inside the room. Thus for the most part, a woman in labor probably still relied on other people to assist her by holding her waist. Once the birth attendants held her waist from behind to support her, it meant that the woman in labor was about to exert strength. "Holding up the waist," *baoyao* 抱腰, therefore became a standard term in medical texts to express the moment right before delivery, and it was considered complementary to the squatting position. This kind of delivery position was still in use during the Song, and may have been the most common position prior to the twentieth century, both in China and abroad.[63]

[63] Zhu Duanzhang, *Weisheng jiabao chanke beiyao*, 6.67 quoting *Yushi beichan jiyongfang* 虞氏備產濟用方: "Although the laboring woman's abdomen might hurt a lot, she must allow others to support her and continuously move without stopping. If bent over, she must be pulled up straight and made to walk from time to time ... wait until the child is pressing to be born, only then allow her to squat." Squatting was still considered best in the Qing dynasty. See Charlotte Furth, "Concepts of Pregnancy, Childbirth and Infancy in Ch'ing Dynasty China," *Journal of Asian Studies* 46.1 (1987): 7-35. Taiwanese women in the Japanese colonial period also squatted down to deliver their children in a "childbirth bucket" or on straw. The childbirth bucket was part of the dowry, and childbirth straw refers to rice straw spread out evenly on the ground. See

Even though a squatting delivery is conducive to exerting strength, if it lasts for too long, the woman in labor runs the danger of exhausting herself. Moreover, holding up her waist also required energy, so the helpers might need to take turns. If she becomes exhausted, the woman in labor might have to lie down to give birth in the supine position. In cases when a woman was lying down, sometimes it must have been on the ground and sometimes in a bed. Yang Zijian's *Shichanlun* explained that in all cases of managing childbirth complications, whether breech or upside-down presentation, sideways (shoulder first) or stalled labor, one should first "make the mother lie down in her bed." This shows that when there were no complications in labor, the woman did not usually lie in bed. In ancient China, from the pre-imperial period to the third century, most people usually sat on mats on the floor, but furniture for lying down did exist, namely, an elevated bed for sleeping. For this reason, Chen Yanzhi described the ancient way of delivery as women "getting down on

---

Yu Chien-ming 游鑑明, "Riju shiqi Taiwan de chanpo" 日據時期台灣的產婆, *Jindai Zhongguo funüshi yanjiu* 近代中國婦女史研究 1 (1993): 49-80. The Hong Kong Chinese include a bucket called "descendants bucket" in a woman's dowry, which might also be related to the squatting position of delivery. See He Hanwei (Hou-wai Ho) 何漢威, ed., *Bendi huaren chuantong hunsu* 本地華人傳統婚俗 (Hongkong: Xianggang Shizhengju, 1986), 32. Until the recent past, Japanese also mostly gave birth by squatting. There was a record for "holding up the waist" is dating from the Heian period (794-1183). In some remote villages people also assumed a delivery position of leaning upright against stairs in response to childbirth complications. See Nakayama Tarō 中山太郎, "Godai no bunbenhō to minzoku" 古代の分娩法と民俗 (Tokyo: Paru tosasha, 1941), 272-94. Women in Western Europe until the recent past also gave birth mostly in vertical positions, such as squatting, crouching, standing, and sitting. See Jacques Gélis, *History of Childbirth: Fertility, Pregnancy and Birth in Early Modern Europe* (Cambridge: Polity Press, 1991), 121-33. Holding up the waist to assist in childbirth is reflected in visual form from antiquity to the present, in China and abroad. In the Dazu stone carving "Shuofumu enzhongjing" 說父母恩重經 (On the enormous grace of one's parents), presumably completed in the Southern Song, the woman in labor in the section of "the grace of suffering in delivery" is standing upright, supported by one woman holding her up from behind from her armpits while another woman kneels down in front of her to receive the newborn (Fig. 3). A terracotta figure from sixth-century BCE Greece also shows a birth assistant holding the waist from behind. See Hilary Bourdillon, *Women as Healers: A History of Women and Medicine* (Cambridge: Cambridge University Press, 1988), 7. In the 1980s, the French obstetrician Michel Odent proposed a new model for giving birth (or it could be called reviving the ancient fashion) that also included holding the waist to assist the woman in labor to give birth squatting. See Michel Odent, *Birth Reborn*, 48. "Holding up the waist" and delivering in the squatting position can be called two aspects of the same thing.

the ground and sitting on straw."[64] In the early imperial period, the four centuries before the Tang dynasty, the shape and usage of beds changed considerably.[65] Sometimes a stool was needed to climb into the bed; the *Xusoushenji* 續搜神記 (Continued records of searching for spirits) recorded that "Wang Meng 王蒙 was only three *chi* 尺 tall and seemingly without bones; when climbing into bed he had to ask people to lift him up."[66] Descending from the bed without the use of a stool or bench is referred to in the histories as "throwing oneself from the bed to the ground," or "throwing oneself down from the bed." During the Southern Dynasties, Xu Xiaosi's 徐孝嗣 mother threw herself from the bed to the ground in an attempt to abort a fetus, illustrating that some beds for sleeping must have been of considerable height.[67] Given the scarcity of information, it is difficult to determine whether it was due to the inconvenience caused by the height of the bed that delivery in the supine position was carried out by spreading a mat and lying on the ground rather than in bed, and the bed was used only after delivery for resting and recuperating or in cases of complications.[68]

---

64 At that time, beds might have been fairly high. The text "Zajinfang" 雜禁方 excavated from Mawangdui recorded that "for frequent nightmares, paint a seven-foot square under the bed." See Ma Jixing, *Mawangdui guyishu kaoshi*, 1008. Ma Jixing explains that "those who tended to suffer from nightmares in their sleep should take seven feet of earth from the ground and smear it below the bed," but it is unclear what the precise activity entailed. Zhou Yimou and Xiao Zuotao, *Mawangdui yishu kaozhu*, 410-11, does not annotate this sentence but explains the method of "smearing a square of five feet [of earth] on top of a well" to prevent dogs from barking in the same text as "spreading five feet [of earth] in a square on top of the well," expressing the idea of warding off. If it did indeed refer to a method for restraining, as Zhou and Xiao explain, and one had to paint the thing to be restrained on top of the well or below the bed in a space of several feet, then beds must have been fairly high at that time.

65 See Qu Xuanying 瞿宣穎, *Zhongguo shehui shiliao congchao jiajizhongce* 中國社會史料叢鈔甲集中冊 (1937; reprint, Taipei: Taiwan Commercial Press, 1965), 260-63 for a discussion on the use of the sitting-beds in the Six Dynasties. For recent research on chairs and beds in early imperial China, see John Kieshnick, *The Impact of Buddhism on Chinese Material Culture* (Princeton: Princeton University Press, 2003), 222-49.

66 *Taiping yulan*, 378.4a.

67 See Li Yanshou, *Nanshi* 南史 (Beijing: Zhonghua shuju, 1975), 15.428; and Ouyang Xiu 歐陽修 and Song Qi 宋祁, *Xin Tangshu* 新唐書 (Beijing: Zhonghua shuju, 1975), 76.3468.

68 Western researchers of childbirth culture suspect that, in the past, women might not have wanted to give birth on the clean and soft bed because they might have been the ones who would need to clean up the big mess afterwards and were therefore willing "to get on the ground and sit on straw." See Edward Shorter, *A History*

If women did give birth by squatting rather than lying in bed, substances discharged during delivery might flow on to the ground. Spreading grass and sprinkling ashes were probably the most frequently used ways of keeping it dry and clean.[69] The expression "sitting on straw" originated from this. Exactly how thick the straw and rushes would have been is difficult to know, but the advice from *Waitai miyao* to "spread a blanket below, for fear that the child will fall on the straw and get hurt" shows that it was probably not too thick. If the day of birth fell on a prohibition day, it would be necessary to have a wild animal skin in addition to straw and ashes. The *Chanjing* said:

> As for [taboo days of] *fanzhi* 反支 (opposing the branch), the spirit comes around and injures people and is called *fanzhi*. When women give birth, if they transgress against it, they will definitely die. One must never be inattentive. If the birth occurs in a month of *fanzhi* it should happen on a cow skin; if it is on ashes, do not let the polluted water or blood or evil substances touch the ground. If they touch the ground, then it will kill people. Again, as for washing and cleaning, in all cases contain everything in a vessel until after this taboo month has passed.[70]

The *Waitai miyao* also pointed out if one let blood or lochia pollute the ground on a tabooed month, it would cause "the child to die in the womb or the birth to not go smoothly." Therefore one must "first spread straw and ashes, and then lay down the skin of a horse,

---

of Women's Bodies (New York: Basic Books, 1982), 56-57. Other scholars suggest that, in addition to convenience, a vertical birth, whether squatting, crouching, standing, or sitting, allowed for more freedom of movement than the horizontal supine position and gave women a greater feeling of participation and importance in their labor. See Gélis, *History of Childbirth*, 121-33.

[69] The use of straw in ancient times included cleaning, for example, the privy. See *Taiping yulan*, 186.7a, quoting Liu Yiqing's 劉義慶 (403-444) *Youming lu* 幽明錄 "When Yu Jin, a Jiande civilian, went to use the toilet, there was always a person who would hand him straw." *Qianjinfang*, 2.31, also recorded treatment for childbirth complications that involved "straw that was used in the privy."

[70] *Ishinpo*, 23.5a. That *fanzhi* were considered tabooed was actually a custom since the pre-imperial period. Both the "Daybook" excavated among the Qin slips from the Yunmeng area 雲夢秦簡日書 and *Hou Hanshu* mention such days. See Yunmeng Shuihudi Qinmu bianjixiaozu 雲夢睡虎地秦墓編輯小組, ed., *Yumeng Shuihudi Qinmu* 雲夢睡虎地秦墓 (Beijing: Wenwu chubanshe, 1981), the back of slips numbers 742, 743. Also Fan Ye 范曄 (398-445), *Hou Hanshu* 後漢書 (Beijing: Zhonghua shuju, 1965), 1640. Also see discussion in Rao Zongyi 饒宗頤 and Zeng Xiantong 曾憲通, *Yunmeng Qinjian rishu yanjiu* 雲夢秦簡日書研究 (Hong Kong: Xianggang zhongwen daxue chubanshe, 1982) (no page numbers), section on "*fanzhi*."

donkey, or cow. Giving birth on top of it will be auspicious."[71] From the various suggestions in the medical texts, one can see people's extreme fear around the time of delivery. Using a cow skin or ashes to deal with the blood and fluid, and catching the water used for cleaning the birthing woman's clothing in a container, and not letting it touch the ground were based on the fear that breaking the prohibitions would offend the spirits with the blood, fluids, and lochia of childbirth. In fact, breaking a taboo was one of the primary reasons employed by people to explain childbirth complications.[72] Medical texts between the sixth and eighth centuries also revealed other explanations for childbirth complications. One was misjudgment by the woman in labor and her assistants regarding the beginning of delivery, with the result of attempting, and failing, to speed up labor.

b) *Problems in Attending Childbirth*

When the child hurt in the mother's womb, this apparently was the sign of impending birth, but the responses by doctors, the woman in labor, and her assistants might have differed on the time to finally squat down and push with force. Wang Shuhe's *Maijing* 脈經 (Canon of the meridians) said, "When a woman is pregnant, her pulses become irregular and floating; if her abdominal pain causes her waist and spine to ache, she is now about to give birth."[73] Again, "When a woman is about to give birth, her pulses become irregular; if she feels [pain] in the middle of the night [according to the *Qianjinfang* the feeling is pain], she will give birth in the middle of the day." Therefore, the manifestation of the pulse was used in conjunction with the sensation of pain to judge the progress during labor.

As soon as the woman in labor experienced pain, assistants might have given her all sorts of things to hold, including, "the fur of a flight-born [flying squirrel]," a sophora branch, or even the head of a cormorant.[74] Holding things might have offered her a place to exert force during labor pains, but the names, shapes, and special

[71] See *Waitai miyao,* 33.927, quoting "Cuishi nianli chengtufa."

[72] *Bingyuanlun*, 43.2-5. "All symptoms of women's childbirth-related disorders" contained all types of explanations for childbirth complications, none of which excluded the possibility of having broken a taboo.

[73] Wang Shuhe, *Maijing* 9.2a.

[74] Recipes from *Xiaopinfang*, quoted from *Waitai miyao*, 34.941, 33.933a, and *Ishinpo*, 23.9ab.

features of these things also seem to have suggested the symbolic meaning of accelerating speed. In early imperial China, people believed that the cormorant gave birth to a fetus rather than laying eggs. "The fetus emerges from the mouth, like a rabbit spitting out a baby; thus when a woman in labor holds it, it facilitates birth."[75] The flying squirrel called "flight-born" is so named because it "gives birth while fly-walking and its baby follows it." Holding its fur was therefore believed to have the effect of disinhibiting delivery.[76] The *Xiaopinfang*, moreover, suggested giving the woman a "flight-born pill," composed of flying squirrel, sophora twigs, and the feathers of an arrow from an old crossbow. The arrow feathers also must have carried the meaning of speed.[77]

To bring the delivery to a quick conclusion must have been the general hope of the woman in labor, the birth assistants, and the household. The medicinal powders for making the fetus slippery and assisting in birth were said to have the effect that "the child will be born by dropping to the ground, without any sensation."[78] However, it is only a small step from the idea that "a quick birth is a smooth birth" to the idea that "a smooth birth is a quick birth." Doctors often suspected that the woman in labor and her assistants tended to exert all their strength prematurely, at the first onset of pain, in order to conclude the delivery quickly, thereby causing childbirth complications.

The *Bingyuanlun* explained the various circumstances of childbirth complications, including breech position, transverse position, fetal death in the womb, and maternal death with the fetus still inside, none of which excluded "causing injury by alarming (the mother) early on." In the case of breech presentation, for example, it was said that "when she first feels pain in the abdomen, the time of birth has not yet arrived, and early alarms cause injury, [because] the baby's rotation is not yet complete and it is born by force."[79] Given the modern gynecological count that pregnancy lasts for forty weeks, in the case of a first birth, most fetuses will turn in the uterus into the

---

[75] Li Shizhen, *Bencao gangmu*, 47.66, section on birds, quoted Tao Hongjing's and Chen Cangqi's 陳藏器 theory. It also quoted Zong Shi's 宗奭 words to correct the mistakes of Tao and Chen.

[76] Tang Wanchun, *Xiaopinfang jilu jianzhu*, 114-15, quoting the *Bielu*.

[77] Tang Wanchun, *Xiaopinfang jilu jianzhu*, 114-15.

[78] Recipe from *Xiaopinfang* quoted in *Waitai miyao*, 34.941.

[79] *Bingyuanlun*, 43.3.

head-down feet-up position during the thirty-sixth to thirty-eighth weeks while fetuses of second or later births will begin to turn and enter the birth position only at the onset of labor pains.[80] From this standpoint, the idea of the *Bingyuanlun* that exerting force prematurely when the child has not yet completed its rotation causes breech or transverse presentation is not entirely unfounded. Premature effort could also mean that "the lochia is already used up when the time of birth has not yet arrived, and the fetus becomes withered and parched, causing the child to die in the womb."[81]

In the case of early alarm that caused the laboring woman to exert force prematurely, Chao Yuanfang did not state clearly whether the people who watch for the birth and hold the woman's waist should be held responsible or not. But he also did not rule out the responsibility of the attendants for disorderly childbirth:

> In the case of maternal death with the fetus still inside, taboos might have been broken, or the time of delivery has not yet arrived but early alarm causes injury, or those watch for the birth lose track of the proper order (of delivering) when holding up her waist to support her. All these lead to childbirth complications, causing the fetus to rise and press against the heart, choking and severing the mother, thereby causing death.[82]

Even when the fetus had already been delivered, doctors also thought it possible for accidents to occur when the attendants hastened to pull out the placenta to conclude the delivery.

> In the old prescriptions, if the placenta did not emerge for a long time and one feared that it might harm the child, one would cut the umbilical cord according to the rules and tie it around something. But it also happened that during the delivery the birth attendants were not considerate and careful, and pulled too strongly, breaking the umbilical cord, causing the placenta to rise up against the heart, thereby killing [the mother].[83]

Thus we can see that, when the placenta failed to be delivered after the fetus had emerged, the most common method of the attendants was to cut the umbilical cord, tie it to something, and wait until the placenta emerged naturally. But if the attendants were anxious and careless, they could also cause the mother's death.

---

[80] David Harvey, ed., *Xinshengming: Huaiyun, fenmian, yuying* 新生命：懷孕—分娩—育嬰 (Hong Kong: Xingdao chubanshe, 1980), 62. Translation by Li Yipei 李宜培, based on the English original, *A New Life* (London: Marshall Cavendish Books, 1979).

[81] *Bingyuanlun*, 43.5.

[82] *Bingyuanlun*, 43.4-5.

[83] *Bingyuanlun*, 43.2. For various recipes to treat retained placenta, see Li Jianmin, "Mawangdui hanmu boshu 'yuzang maibaotu' jianzheng," appendix 2, 803-6.

The earliest extant description of childbirth that explained complications in terms of disorderly assistance was Cui Zhiti's quotation recorded in Wang Tao's *Waitai miyao*:

> Now as for death in childbirth, it is most common in wealthy households, where many women live together. Once the fetus begins to turn and she feels pain, the others will be informed immediately. The attendants become anxious and cause her to be startled. Alarm and fright accumulate, thus causing disharmony of her physiological functions and disorder of her *qi*, only increasing her pain. When the attendants see her pain increasing, they think that the time has come. Some might bind her hair in a knot, some might work on her abdomen, and some might wash her face with cold water. They exert great effort to push, and the child emerges suddenly. The accumulated *qi* all of a sudden will gush out below without stopping, to the point that she passes out.[84]

According to Cui Zhiti's account, "childbirth complications to the point of death are unheard of among concubines giving birth secretly or poor maidservants delivering alone." Therefore he suggested that a delivery would run smoothly when "no one was intruding to stand by so that everything was allowed to run its proper course," and complications to the point of death were due to too many people worrying and yelling and assisting in birth inappropriately.[85]

According to doctors, the biggest problem of the laboring woman and her attendants was that they mistakenly believed the pain from the fetus turning in the abdomen to be the fetus pressing forth, wanting to be born. This is why Wang Shuhe pointed out that "if her abdominal pain causes her waist and spine to ache, she is now about to give birth." Chao Yuanfang further clarified the matter, stating that "when the laboring woman's abdomen hurts but not her waist, it is not yet birth. When the pain in the abdomen is linked to the waist and is severe, then it is birth."[86] Cui Zhiti expressed that it was harmful for the delivery if, at the time of birth, the female relatives gathered around, and suggested that, in order to avoid mistakes made in this confusion, it was better if the woman followed the natural order of things by herself (see discussion below). Sun Simiao also warned the family of the woman that "whenever the time of delivery has come, it is particularly prohibited to have many people observe it. Allow two to three people at the most to attend at her side. Only

---

[84] *Waitai miyao*, 33.924, citing Cui Zhiti's quotation from a certain Master Luan.
[85] *Waitai miyao*, 33.924.
[86] *Bingyuanlun*, 43.2-3.

after the birth is completed, inform the others. If crowds of people observe it, there are bound to be childbirth complications."[87]

c) *Treating Childbirth Complications*

A delivery that took too long was a key indication of birth complications. But the woman giving birth, the birth attendants, and the doctors might have had different ideas regarding how long labor had to last before birth complication was considered. Whenever medical texts mentioned a time, they used "several days" or "lasting days" to refer to childbirth complications.[88] There were also instances that specify three days or three to five days.[89] In the *Waitai miyao* birth story in which the delivery is aided by suspending ropes and tying wood to them, the laboring woman's abdominal pains began at *ribu* 日晡 (late afternoon), and the child was finally born at the end of the "fifth night-watch." The doctor recollected the situation as follows:

> At *ribu*, I was told that the woman's abdomen hurt which seemed to be a symptom of birth.... I explained to her the methods, each in due course. This woman seemed to understand my words. After I finished speaking, I ordered the door be closed and set up a bed outside where I sat together with Qing [the woman's father-in-law, who requested the doctor's help], not allowing even one person to enter. From time to time, I asked through the door how things were, and she answered that the pain was slight and bearable. At the first night-watch, I gave orders to thoroughly cook a hen that died of a natural cause, and then to make nonglutinous rice porridge with the soup... I encouraged her to eat about three *sheng* 升.[90] By the end of the fifth night-watch, she gave birth to a child by herself. I did not let people enter until I heard the child's cry. The woman who gave birth was at ease, calm and stable, with nothing out of the ordinary.[91]

The first night watch was from seven to nine o'clock during the night, and the fifth from three to five in the morning.[92] From the

[87] *Qianjinfang*, 2.30.

[88] See medical texts cited in *Waitai miyao*, 33.933ab, 936b, and *Ishinpo*, 23.16b-17a.

[89] See *Qianjinfang*, 2.30-31, and *Ishinpo*, 23.11b.

[90] One *sheng* was about 0.2 liter in early China, but expanded to almost 0.6 liter in the Tang.

[91] *Waitai miyao*, 33.924, citing Cui Zhiti's quotation of a certain Master Luan.

[92] *Bu* 晡 is the hours of *shen* 申, between three and five o'clock in the afternoon. It is separated into three periods, early, middle, and late *bu*. The end of *shen* is the last *bu*, when the sun is about to set, often referred to as *ribu* in historical texts. For a discussion

tone of the description, the doctor seemed to have considered that twelve hours passing from the time the pregnant woman experienced abdominal pain to the birth of the child was a fairly smooth and normal delivery. Maybe the "three days" mentioned in the medical literature signified the point when doctors felt that the life of the mother was endangered, the time limit when intervention became necessary. Between twelve hours and three days, doctors might have disagreed on the degree of intervention called for. And when they did enter to assist in childbirth, they would try to shorten the time with all sorts of treatments, including medical prescriptions, invocations, and ritual acts.

For childbirth complications, there were all sorts of birth-hastening herbal prescriptions in the medical texts which mostly contained mallow seed, dianthus, angelica, achyranthes, typha pollen, ligusticum, licorice, and so forth. Some were brewed in liquor while some were fried in pig lard and then ingested in liquor. The characteristic of mallow seed was considered slippery and disinhibiting, able to make the fetus slippery, as discussed earlier.[93] All medical texts stated that dianthus disinhibited discharge below, thus, for example, freeing urination and blocked blood, as well as having the special property of eliminating purulence.[94] Angelica regulated the blood and had been an important gynecological herb since ancient times.[95] Achyranthes was said to precipitate static blood,[96] and Tao Hongjing stated that typha pollen also had the effect of purifying blood.[97] Ligusticum was indicated for all sorts of headache, and its

of time indicators, see Gu Yanwu 顧炎武 (1613-82), *Rizhilu* 日知錄 (Taipei: Minglun shuju, 1971), 21.576-79, the entry on "*gu wu yiri fenwei shier shi*" 古無一日分爲十二時; Zhou Yiliang 周一良, *Wei Jin Nanbeichao shi zhaji* 魏晉南北朝史札記 (Beijing: Zhonghua shuju, 1985), 135-37.

[93] For recipes using mallow seeds to treat complications, see *Qianjinfang*, 2.31, 32, 33; *Waitai miyao*, 33.935, 937; *Ishinpo*, 23.11b, 13b, 18a.

[94] For recipes using dianthus to treat complications, see *Qianjinfang*, 2, 31, 32; *Waitai miyao*, 33.935, 937b; *Ishinpo*, 23.11b, 34ab. On dianthus, the *Bielu* stated: "Dianthus grows in the mountain valleys of Taishan;" Su Song: "It is now available everywhere." *Bencao Gangmu*, "Herbs," 16.107-8.

[95] For recipes using angelica, see *Qianjinfang*, 2. 32; *Waitai miyao*, 33. 937b; *Ishinpo*, 23.11b-12a.

[96] For recipes using achyranthes, see *Qianjinfang*, 2, 30-32; *Waitai miyao*, 33.937b; *Ishinpo*, 23.16b, 18a, 34b. The *Bencao gangmu* recorded that "*Bielu* stated: 'Achyranthes grows in river valleys east of the Yellow River and Linqu 臨朐. Su Song added: 'Now it is also available in the area between the Yangtze and Huai Rivers, as well as in Min 閩 and Yue 粵.'" See *Bencao gangmu*, "Herbs," 16.79-82.

[97] For recipes using typha pollen to treat complications, see *Qianjinfang*, 2.32; *Waitai*

most important effect for the suffering mother during a drawn-out delivery was perhaps to settle the spirit.[98] According to Zhen Quan (540-643), licorice "treats seventy-two types of mammary rock poison, resolves the twelve hundred kinds of toxics from herbs and trees, and harmonizes the effects of all medicines."[99] Tao Hongjing stated, "This herb is the ruler of all herbs; there are few classic prescriptions that do not use it."[100] In addition, there were recipes for ingesting all sorts of large and small legumes,[101] chicken eggs,[102] and mercury. Mercury, being a deadly poison, was sometimes used in recipes for abortion, but, in most cases, doctors did not encourage its use in treating complications.[103] Swallowing chicken eggs was believed to preserve the woman's strength during labor, and, similar to swallowing sesame oil, to aid in delivery by making the fetus slippery, due to the eggs' slimy consistency.

The extant medical literature of early imperial China contains numerous herbal recipes for treating childbirth complications. Moreover, the explanations of the origins of each herb by Tao Hongjing from the Six Dynasties period, Su Gong 蘇恭 from the Tang, and Su Song 蘇頌 from the Northern Song show that between the fifth and the tenth centuries, the cultivation area of many medicinally used herbs increased continuously, whether because of increased trade or cultural exchange.[104] When it was impossible to obtain

miyao, 33.932b, 936b, 937b; *Ishinpo*, 23.13a. Typha pollen is the stamen of fragrant typha. The *Bencao gangmu* recorded that "*Bielu* states: 'Typha pollen stems from the lakes and marshes east of the Yellow River.' Su Song added: 'It is available everywhere; the best stems [come] from Qin.'" See *Bencao gangmu*, "Herbs," 19.98-101.

[98] For recipes using ligusticum to treat complications, see *Waitai miyao*, 33.936b; *Ishinpo*, 23.13b, 16a. The *Bencao gangmu* recorded that "*Bielu* stated: 'The leaves of ligusticum are called *miwu* 蘼蕪. It grows in river valleys in Wugong 武功 and on the western slopes of the Xie valley.' Tao Hongjing stated: 'Wugong and the western slopes of the Xie Valley are all near Changan. Now in Liyang 歷陽 many people cultivate it everywhere.' Su Song added: 'It is common in the mountains of Shanxi, Shannxi, Sichuan, and east of the Yangtze River.'" See *Bencao gangmu*, "Herbs," 14. 5-7.

[99] Cited in *Bencao gangmu*, "Herbs," 12.81.

[100] For recipes using licorice to treat complications, see *Qianjinfang*, 2.32; *Waitai miyao*, 33.935-36; *Ishinpo*, 22.34a, 23.16b-17a. Also see *Bencao gangmu*, "Herbs," 12.81-85.

[101] For recipes on ingesting legumes to treat complications, see *Qianjinfang*, 2.31; *Waitai miyao*, 33.933a, 937b; *Ishinpo*, 22.34ab, 35a, 23.11b, 12b, 13a, 18b.

[102] For recipes using chicken eggs, see *Qianjinfang*, 2.31; *Waitai miyao*, 33.932b, 935ab, 936b; *Ishinpo*, 23.13a, 18a, 34ab.

[103] *Bencao gangmu*, "Stones," 9.56-59.

[104] The increase in the growing areas and circulation of medicinal herbs raise

certain medicinal herbs and in cases in which medicinal herbs were considered insufficient, doctors suggested other kinds of treatments, for example, heat application and massage, sneezing and vomiting, and pushing the fetus back to be born again.

In terms of the applying heat and massage, one recipe advised using "three *sheng* of earth from an ant hill, boil it until hot, contain it in a bag and drag it over the area below the heart."[105] Another recommendation was to "apply cow manure to the mother's abdomen," or to "rub salt on the mother's abdomen." [106] Another was to "boil peach root down to a thick liquid and use it to bathe her below the knees."[107] The Tibetan *Zaliaofang* 藏醫雜療方 (Tibetan recipes of various remedies) unearthed at Dunhuang suggested using the tail of either a roe deer or a deer, crushed and pounded, and spread on the woman's vagina. Alternatively, the horn of a wild buffalo or antelope combined with the dirt from a 'stallion's whip' might be applied to the laboring woman's hipbone.[108] It even advocated that the laboring woman mount an ox's saddle while a strong man pushed down hard on her shoulders.[109] Since sneezing and vomiting encourage the abdominal muscles to contract, birth assistants might have inserted gleditsia in the nose to make the laboring woman sneeze, or they might have tickled her throat with hair to make her vomit, assuming that might help expel the placenta.[110] Because women sometimes experience nausea at the onset of labor, it is also possible that the assistants interpreted vomiting as the fetus pressing, wanting to

interesting and complex questions. For example, how could a household during the Southern Dynasties obtain herbs from the north or the northwest, such as angelica, achyranthes, cattail pollen, ligusticum, and other herbs mentioned in the *Sengshenfang* or *Xiaopinfang*, texts composed and circulating during that time? Were they sold for a high price, or substituted for with cheaper local products? Did people employ alternative ritual or manual treatment methods because herbs were difficult to obtain? Although these questions are significant, it is impossible to answer them given the currently available information.

[105] *Xiaopinfang* cited in *Ishinpo*, 23.16b. See *Qianjinfang*, 2.33 for a similar recipe.

[106] *Xiaopinfang* and *Wenzhongfang* 文仲方, cited in *Waitai miyao*, 33.934ab, 936b; *Geshifang* 葛氏方, cited in *Ishinpo*, 23.14a; *Qianjinfang*, 2.31.

[107] *Lungmenfang* 龍門方, cited in *Ishinpo*, 23.16a.

[108] The term "whip" *bian* 鞭 could also mean the penis of the male animals.

[109] P.T. 1057 (P.T. is the representative code of Paul Pelliat's Tibetan documents kept in the Bibliothè-que Nationale de Paris), annotated translation in Wang Yao 王堯 and Chen Jian 陳踐, *Dunhuang Tufan wenxianxuan* 敦煌吐蕃文獻選 (Chengdu: Sichuan minzu chubanshe, 1983), 174.

[110] *Xiaopinfang*, cited in *Ishinpo*, 23.17b. Also see *Waitai miyao*, 33.937a.

be born. Based on this reasoning, the medical texts frequently recorded such emetic methods as forcing the laboring woman to drink vinegar, water containing charred straw used in the privy, her husband's urine, or other such substances.[111] If such methods did have an effect, it may have been that they made the laboring woman feel like vomiting and thus stimulated the contractions.

The conditions for which herbs were most rarely employed were breech and adverse presentation, probably because the doctors feared that birth-accelerating medicines would not only fail to facilitate birth but would "make the child rise and press against the heart," endangering the mother. Therefore, physically therapeutic methods instead of herbal medicines were often applied. In addition to massaging the mother's abdomen, other methods were used to make the child return in the womb so that the process of birth could be started all over again. These included applying salt, powder, pure cinnabar, black soot, or cart grease to the fetus's soles or under the armpits, or pinching it tightly.[112] The method for poking with a needle, described in the *Xiaopinfang*, contained the most detail:

> A method to treat breech and lateral presentation, or when the hands and feet emerge first: One can take a thick needle and poke the child's hands and feet, entering about two *fen* 分. Feeling pain, the child will turn around in fright and then contract, naturally rotating to the ideal position.[113]

In addition, medical texts also recorded many ritual actions to treat childbirth complications. Among them, "to open doors, windows, pitchers, kettles and all sorts of covered things" expresses people's belief in the mutual correspondence between things, that is, they assumed that opening some sort of external object would be beneficial for opening the Gate of Birth.[114] Sometimes, medicinal preparations included aspects of ritual behavior, such as the rule to use "eastward-flowing water" and an "east-facing stove" to boil the herbs.[115] Sometimes ritual behavior was accompanied by invocations and written charms. The characters were written on cracked soybeans,

---

[111] See recipes of *Xiaopinfang*, cited in *Ishinpo*, 23.16a, and *Qianjinfang*, 2.30-33.

[112] See recipes of *Xiaopinfang* and *Jiyanfang*, cited in *Waitai miyao*, 33.934 and *Ishinpo*, 23.13b. According to Ma Jixing, "Yixinfang zhong de guyixue wenxian chutan," *Jiyanfang* was written by Yao Sengyuan 姚僧垣 of the Northern Zhou dynasty (557-81).

[113] *Xiaopinfang*, cited in *Waitai miyao*, 33.935a. One *fen* equals to one-tenth of a body inch.

[114] *Chanjing*, cited in *Ishinpo*, 23.11b.

[115] *Jiyanfang*, cited in *Waitai miyao*, 33.935-36; also cited in *Ishinpo*, 23.16b-17a.

peach kernels, or the soles of the baby's feet in cases of breech or adverse presentation.[116] The laboring mother might be asked to hold an inscribed object in her hand, to swallow it whole or charred into ashes in water.[117] In addition to special talismanic characters, the text contains such individual characters as "day," "moon," "thousand," "black," "fine," "exit," or sentences like "quickly come out, quickly come out," "emerge the placenta and the child, do not cause illness for the mother," or the name of the child's father, showing that people believed in the magical power of writing.[118]

Birth was understood as the result of sex between men and women and, among the various treatments of childbirth complications, peculiar recipes related to male or female gender also appeared, such as charring menstrual cloth and letting the woman in labor ingest it.[119] While pregnancy and delivery were women's business, recipes for birth assistance also reflected the idea of the husband's responsibility. For instance, to cover up the well with the husband's clothes (especially his underwear) would cause the fetus and placenta to "emerge at once." It was "excellent" to char a belt from the husband's trousers into ashes and have the woman in labor ingest it in liquor. If the laboring woman drank one or two *sheng* of the husband's urine, it helped to expel a dead fetus. Ingesting the husband's fingernails, charred and ground into powder, or his pubic hair, dry-roasted and then mixed with cinnabar paste, to be swallowed by the laboring woman, could treat breech and adverse presentation. The characters of the husband's name, written on the child's soles, could cause a smooth delivery. The husband should bring wa-

---

[116] *Chanjing*, cited in *Ishinpo*, 23.11b-12a; *Geshifang*, cited in *Ishinpo*, 23.14a; *Shanfanfang* 刪繁方, cited in *Waitai miyao*, 33.934b-35a.

[117] *Xiaopinfang*, cited in *Waitai miyao*, 33.933b, 937a; *Shanfanfang*, cited in *Waitai miyao*, 33.934b-35a; *Chanjing*, cited in *Ishinpo*, 23.11b, 17a-b.

[118] *Jiyanfang*, cited in *Ishinpo*, 23.13b; also see *Qianjinfang*, 2.32.

[119] *Geshifang*, cited in *Ishinpo*, 23.17b. In addition, retained placenta was also treated by giving the laboring woman a charred kitchen apron or bamboo bowl to ingest, such as suggested by the *Jiyanfang*, cited in *Waitai miyao*, 33.937b. Both of these were important tools used by women in their everyday household chores. The symbolic significance of medical recipes that called for charring, pulverizing, and ingesting such objects to treat childbirth complications was not limited to sex as such, but also extended to women's gender roles in society. For discussion of the efficacy of gendered body parts in medicine, see Li Zhende (Jen-der Lee), "Han-Tang zhijian yifang zhongde jijian furen yu nüti weiyao," 漢唐之間醫方中的忌見婦人與女體爲藥, *Xinshixue* 新史學 13.4 (2002): 1-36.

ter from outside in his mouth and put it in his wife's mouth, and if performed a thousand times, "a difficult fetus will emerge immediately." Numerous examples of this kind illustrated the weight of the husband's role.[120]

Delivery by opening the abdomen surgically was completely absent from medical literature of early imperial China. Recorded in the marvel stories from the Six Dynasties were several accounts of children being born from under the armpits or the flanks, expressing that people did have an idea about birth by opening the abdomen, but it is doubtful that this can be seen as evidence for cutting open a living person to take out the fetus.[121] Considering the story of a certain Ms. Lin from the fifth century, it appears that Caesarean section, if ever performed, could only be done if the pregnant woman had already died. The *Yiyuan* 異苑 (Garden of wonders) said:

> Ms. Lin, wife of Wu Biao in the country of Pei沛 was pregnant, fell ill, and died in the era of Yuanjia (424-53). Because the local custom considered it a taboo to bury a woman with a fetus, they had to cut her open to remove it. The wife's wet nurse felt so terribly sad that she cursed [the heaven] while stroking the corpse: "If there is indeed a Heaven's Way, do not allow her to be cut up after death." All of a sudden, the corpse's face took on pink color, and [the wet nurse] called the servants to prop her up. Immediately the child dropped to the ground and the corpse fell over."[122]

Whether Ms. Lin was spared the fate of being cut up as a corpse because "there is indeed a Heaven's Way," or whether she had in

---

[120] See recipes from *Xiaopinfang*, *Sengshenfang*, *Jiyanfang* and *Chanjing*, cited in *Ishinpo*, 23.11b, 12ab, 13b, 14a, 16a, 18a; *Jiyanfang*, *Guangjifang*, *Shanfanfang*, and *Qianjinfang*, cited in *Waitai miyao*, 33.934b, 935a, 936b; also see the Tibetan medical recipe in P.T. 1057, annotated translation in Wang Yao and Chen Jian, *Dunhuang Tufan wenxianxuan*, 174.

[121] *Taiping yulan*, 361.5a, quoting *Xuanzhongji* 玄中記, recorded the birth of a child from the back flanks; 361.7b, quoting the *Liexianzhuan* 列仙傳, recorded Laozi's 老子 mother cutting her left armpit to give birth to Laozi, obviously a mythological story. But in the *Sanguozhi Weizhi* 三國志魏志, recorded in the Huangchu period (220-26), a certain Ms. Wang delivered a boy who emerged from her right armpit. It said that, "The boy's mother is self-possessed and without extraordinary pain. Now her wounds are already healed, mother and child are stable and safe, without calamities or harm." Ma Dazheng regards it as very likely that this was indeed a Caesarean section. He also quotes a story from Fang Xuanling 房玄齡 (578-648), *Jinshu* 晉書 (Beijing: Zhonghua shuju, 1974), 97.2542, saying a certain Ms. An from the region in the west, "in the twelfth month of pregnancy, delivered a child by cutting open the flanks" as a proof that Caesarean section was practiced when pregnancy was overdue. See Ma Dazheng, *Zhongguo fuchanke fazhanshi*, 68.

[122] *Taiping yulan*, 361.9b.

fact not yet died completely and the wet-nurse revived her when she stroked the corpse, is unknowable and involves the standards and capabilities for determining death at that time.[123] Since a woman with complications in childbirth might have suddenly passed out and stayed unconscious for quite a while, it might have been difficult for the attendants to determine whether she was dead or alive. Medical texts like the *Jiyanfang* 集驗方 (Recipes of collected efficacies) and the *Bingyuanlun* instructed the birth assistants on how to judge the situation:

> Symptoms for life or death in childbirth complications: If the mother's face is red and her tongue green, the child is dead and the mother alive. If her lips and mouth are green and she is salivating from both sides of the mouth, both mother and child are dead; if her face is green and the tongue red and she is salivating, the mother is dead and the child alive."[124]

If the child was dead and the mother alive, it was probably treated according to the methods to remove a dead fetus in the abdomen. But if the child and mother had both died and there was no taboo against putting her in a coffin with a fetus inside, then were the mother and child buried together? And if the mother was dead and the child alive, were there times when the abdomen was cut open to remove the fetus? Because of the scarcity of historical information, it is difficult to know clearly; one cannot help but wonder.[125]

Postpartum

When the fetus was born and the placenta delivered, the major task of the birth was done, but it was still not completely over.

---

[123] In marvel stories and histories from the Six Dynasties, there were many accounts of women dying in childbirth and the child afterwards being born inside the tomb. These stories raise questions about contemporary capability in determining death.

[124] *Ishinpo*, 23.10b, quoting the *Yimenfang* and *Jiyanfang*. Only the quotation "if her face is red and her tongue green and she is salivating, the mother is dead and the child alive" disagrees with *Bingyuanlun*, 43, which records that "when the face is green, the tongue red, and she is salivating, the mother is dead and the child alive." According to Ma Jixing, "Yixinfang zhong de guyixue wenxian chutan," the *Yimenfang* was composed in the Tang or before.

[125] Accounts of children being born inside tombs were not that rare and showed that people in that time believed that a woman could give birth after her death. In this light, people of the early imperial period might have had different ideas regarding the borderline between life and death.

In addition to taking care of the newborn, washing it and cutting the umbilical cord, the birth attendants also had to pay attention to the mother's condition. Modern Chinese medicine divides the postpartum time into the two periods of "recently delivered" and "lying-in," the former indicating the first seven days after delivery and the latter from delivery to the point when the mother's reproductive organs have recovered to their normal condition, usually about six to eight weeks.[126] In the medical literature in early imperial China, the various problems after delivery were all referred to as postpartum disorders, *chanhoubing* 產後病. As to what period the term "postpartum" referred to, expressions in the medical texts ranged from three days, seven days, thirty days, a full month, one hundred days, and half a year up to as long as a whole year.[127] In fact, after undergoing childbirth, a woman's physical constitution was changed, and she could potentially suffer all sorts of symptoms for the rest of her life. A few conditions that arose soon after delivery and could have been life-threatening were treated differently from the usual long-term medical care and physical hygiene practices of supplementing deficiencies. In the following, I will discuss the management of postpartum problems in two aspects, namely, emergency care and health preservation.

a) *Risks Immediately After Delivery*

After the child was born and the placenta delivered, most likely the mother would be carried to a cleaner place to rest. The straw bedding used for delivery was disposed of by burning. The *Taichanshu* from Mawangdui stated that giving the newborn a bath in water mixed with the burnt straw bedding could prevent it from contracting skin diseases. Giving the mother half a cup of the water in which the newborn had been bathed would ensure that "the mother will also have no other illnesses."[128] To preserve the mother's emotional balance immediately after delivery, the *Chanjing* suggested, "Right after a woman gives birth to a child, do not allow her to observe

[126] Luo Yuankai 羅元愷, ed., *Zhongyi fukexue* 中醫婦科學 (Taipei: Zhiyin chubanshe, 1989), 260.

[127] For different ideas and expressions about the postpartum period, see *Bingyuanlun*, 43.9; *Qianjinfang*, 3.36-37; *Jiyanfang*, *Guangjifang*, and *Jiujifang* 救急方, cited in *Waitai miyao*, 34.944a, 947b-948a, 953a.

[128] Ma Jixing, *Mawangdui guyishu kaoshi*, 812.

herself. As for the people beside her, none of them may ask about the gender."[129] The *Qianjinfang* also stated, "When the child has completely emerged, all people, including the mother, are forbidden to ask whether it is a girl or a boy."[130] While the medical literature before the Tang did not explain the reasoning behind this practice, Song doctors pointed out that its goal was to avoid influencing the mother's emotions if the newborn's gender did not fulfill her hopes.[131] This practice was the exact opposite of the advice given in the Tibetan medical documents excavated in Dunhuang: "After the child is born, make it sleep in the mother's embrace."[132] In addition, the *Qianjinfang* stated, "Do not let the mother see the filth and pollution."[133] The medical texts acknowledged the laboring woman's pollution straightforwardly and advised the family to avoid other polluting sources: "When birth is impending, or after it is concluded, never allow people from a mourning household to enter in. If they observe labor or delivery, there will be complications in birth or, if the birth is already over, it will harm the child."[134]

Medical texts also paid special attention to caring for the mother's physical health. The *Qianjinfang* pointed out, "One must worry not only when a woman is about to deliver a child, one must exercise extreme caution at the postpartum stage."[135] In order to prevent blood dizziness or blood counter-flowing, Song doctors recommended that for three days after delivery women should "stay in bed propped up high, and lie on the back with the knees up."[136] No such rules were found in the medical texts before the Tang, but they also tended to employ three days as a time limit. According to the *Xiaopinfang*:

> There are three days of life and death. In the old times, when women gave birth by getting down on the ground and sitting on straw, this was just like awaiting death. If she did survive and give birth, this was called "escaping the adversity." The relatives all brought pig liver to congratulate her. It was

[129] *Ishinpo*, 23.25a.
[130] *Qianjinfang*, 2.30.
[131] Chen Ziming, *Furen daquan liangfang*, 18.485.
[132] Tibetan medical recipe in P.T.1057, annotated translation in Wang Yao and Chen Jian, *Dunhuang Tufan wenxianxuan*, 174.
[133] *Qianjinfang*, 3.30.
[134] *Qianjinfang*, 3.30.
[135] *Qianjinfang*, 3.30.
[136] *Furen daquan liangfang*, 18.485.

to replenish and nurture her damaged five internal [organs], not to celebrate the child."[137]

The greatest concern for a woman's safety after delivery was to prevent the illnesses of blood dizziness and convulsion sickness. The *Bingyuanlun* distinguished the postpartum *qi* depression of blood dizziness into two kinds, excessive blood loss and insufficient discharge of blood, and points out that, "If vexatious depression does not stop, it will kill her."[138] Other medical literature of the early imperial period describes the symptoms of blood dizziness as heart depression with *qi* collapse, inability to open the eyes, loss of consciousness, and inability to wake up.[139]

To arouse the mother, medical texts suggested pouring cold water in her face or yanking her hair and knees.[140] To stimulate her with smells, vinegar or liquor might be rubbed in her mouth and nose, or someone might spit in her face, or urine, birth blood, or even horse manure forced down her throat.[141] One recipe called for ingesting the newborn's bath water, similar to the above-mentioned suggestion in the *Taichanshu*.[142] The management of blood dizziness and the treatment of childbirth complications were identical in that they both contained numerous physical therapeutic methods. As for the herbs applied, the most important one in emergency care was rehmannia, which was usually indicated for uterine bleeding. Whether used in fresh or dried form, rehmannia often appeared in medical recipes for the treatment of both hemorrhage with fainting and for lochiorrhea.[143] For instance, the *Yimenfang* 醫門方 (Recipes of the

---

137 *Ishinpo*, 23.25a.

138 *Bingyuanlun*, 43.6.

139 See *Jingxinfang* 經心方, *Jiyanfang*, *Chanjing*, *Qianjinfang*, *Mengshenfang* 孟詵方, and *Zimu milu* 子母秘錄, cited in *Ishinpo*, 23.26a-27a; also *Guangjifang*, *Wenzhongfang*, *Jiuojifang*, *Cuishi*, and *Jinxiaofang* 近效方, cited in *Waitai miyao*, 34.946b-47b.

140 See recipes of *Jiyanfang*, *Qianjinfang*, and *Mengshenfang*, cited in *Ishinpo*, 23.26b-27a; also *Cuishi*, cited in *Waitai miyao*, 34.947b.

141 See recipes of *Jinxinfang*, *Qianjinfang*, and *Yimenfang*, cited in *Ishinpo*, 23.26a-27a; also *Jingxinfang*, *Cuishi*, and *Jinxiaofang*, cited in *Waitai miyao*, 34.947ab.

142 *Cuishi*, cited in *Waitai miyao*, 34.947b.

143 See recipes in *Yimenfang*, *Boji anzhongfang* 博濟安眾方, cited in *Ishinpo*, 23.27a; *Guangjifang*, *Wenzhongfang*, and *Xujenze chanhoufang* 許仁則產後方, cited in *Waitai miyao*, 34.946b-49a, 956b-57a. Also, *Qianjinfang*, 3.40-43. *Bencao gangmu* recorded that "*Bielu* stated: 'Rehmannia that grows in yellow soil of the rivers and marshes of Xianyang 咸陽 is superior.' Tao Hongjing stated: 'The variety from Weicheng 渭城 has seeds like wheat. At present, dried rehmannia from Pengcheng 彭城 is the best, next the one

medical family), section on "recipes for postpartum incessant bleeding" said to "quickly pulverize dried rehmannia, ingest one spoon in liquor, and it will stop after two to three doses." In *Guangjifang* 廣濟方 (Recipes of broad relief), rehmannia was used in combination with other herbs to treat "profuse uterine bleeding, which is incessant, knotting pain in the abdomen, and panting." The descriptions in these two works illustrated most vividly the urgency in a situation of profuse uterine bleeding.[144]

In addition to profuse uterine bleeding, doctors were most concerned with postpartum convulsions, *jing* 痙. The symptoms of convulsions included the teeth being clamped tight shut, the four limbs thrashing, neck and back being straight and stiff, and muscles being difficult to bend, all of which traditional medical texts considered to be caused by contracting Wind cold. The above-mentioned *Wushier bingfang* section on "infant-cord rigidity" explained that it was caused by "remaining on wet ground for too long." Zhang Zhongjing stated that new mothers often suffered from three illnesses, one of them being convulsions, *bingjing* 病痙; another fainting, *bingyumou* 病鬱冒; and the other "difficult defecation."[145] According to him convulsions were caused by contracting cold: "Right after delivery, their blood is deficient, they sweat profusely and they are likely to be struck by Wind,"[146] which constituted a life-threatening danger. The *Bingyuanlun* called it "postpartum Wind-stroke convulsions," *chanhou zhongfengjing* 產後中風痙, and explained that "it is caused by Wind *qi* obtaining entry into the five organs ... again, she contracts cold and dampness, cold strikes the sinews and erupts as convulsions." As soon as convulsions erupted, "the mouth is clenched tightly, the back arched straight; she shakes her head and whinnies like a horse and the waist twisted. It erupts ten times in a moment, her breath-

---

from Liyang. Recently, the one from Jiangning Banqiao 江寧板橋 is most superior.' Su Song stated: 'Now it is available everywhere. It is best to use the one from the Tong province." See *Bencao gangmu*, "Herbs," 13.73-79.

[144] *Yimenfang*, cited in *Ishinpo*, 23.27a; and *Guangjifang*, cited in *Waitai miyao*, 34.948b.

[145] *Jingui yaolue*, 21.307, identical to *Maijing*, 9.7a. The mother's appetite could suffer due to constipation, and, in elite families, if she had been inactive from pre-delivery bed-rest to her postpartum recovery, the situation might have been even worse.

[146] Xu Zhongke commented, "The body is hot and averse to cold, the feet are cold and the face red, the mouth is suddenly clenched, the back arched." *Jingui yaolüe*, 21.307.

ing is urgent to the point of being cut off, her sweating is so profuse like rain that there is not enough time to wipe it with hands. In all these cases, she will die."[147] The *Qianjinfang* described the patient's body being arched back rigidly like a bow bent backward and calls it "childbed Wind," *rufeng* 蓐風. It also warned that "if she resembles a bent bow, her fate is like a flickering candle."[148]

There were a great number of treatments in the medical texts for wind-stroke convulsions. The herbs most frequently used in the drugs included angelica root, fresh or dried ginger, cinnamon bark, puerariae, ovate atractylodes, soybeans, and ledebouriella. Angelica root was called *duhuo* 獨活 in Chinese and was indicated for the various types of wind cold, either made into a decoction or brewed in liquor. According to the medical literature, it could also be used "for people so depleted that they could not ingest other medicines."[149] Gingers, both fresh and dried, were thought to "expel wind and remove dampness."[150] Cinnamon bark was recommended in medical texts for all cases of wind *qi*.[151] Pueraria was indicated for the various paralytic impediments, *bi* 痹, used since the Han to treat cold

---

147 *Bingyuanlun*, 43.15.

148 *Qianjinfang*, 3.40.

149 See recipes of *Geshifang*, *Xiaopinfang*, *Sengshenfang*, *Luyanfang*, *Chanjing*, cited in *Ishinpo*, 23.32b-34b; and *Waitai miyao*, 34.952a-53a. Also see recipe of *Boji anzhongfang*, cited in *Waitai miyao*, 34.958ab; and recipes in *Qianjinfang*, 3.40-43. About Angelica root, the *Bielu* stated: "It grows in the river valleys of Yongzhou 雍州, or in Annan 安南 of the Gansu province." Tao Hongjing stated: "This area is now the Qiang 羌 territory. *Qianghuo* 羌活 is in appearance fine, with many sections, soft and with a strong smell. The herb coming from Xichuan of Northern Yizhou 益州西川 constitutes *duhuo*." Su Song stated: "At present, the *duhuo* and *qianghuo* coming out of Sichuan is the best." For all quotations, see *Bencao gangmu*, "Herbs," 13.49-51.

150 For the medicinal use of fresh and dried gingers, see recipe in *Jingui yaolüe*, 21.313; recipes of *Geshifang*, *Sengshenfang*, *Chanjing*, cited in *Ishinpo*, 23.33a-34b; and *Waitai miyao*, 34.953a. Also see recipes in *Qianjinfang*, 2.40-43. As for gingers, the *Bielu* stated: "Fresh and dried gingers come from the mountain valleys in Jianwei 犍爲 [ancient prefecture in Sichuan], as well as from Jingzhou 荊州 [ancient state of Chu, covering Hunan, most of Hubei, and parts of Guizhou] and Yangzhou 揚州 [ancient province, land south of the Huai and Yangzi rivers, most of modern Jiangxi, Zhejiang, and Fujian]." Su Song stated: "It is available everywhere. The best comes from Han, Wen, and Chizhou 漢溫池州." For all quotations, see *Bencao gangmu*, "Vegetables," 17.72-78.

151 See recipes of *Chanjing*, cited in *Ishinpo*, 23.34b. Also see recipes in *Qianjinfang*, 3.40-43. Regarding the cultivation area of cinnamon, Su Gong stated: "The best quality comes from Rongzhou, 融州 Guizhou 桂州, and Jiaozhou 交州." See *Bencao gangmu*, "Trees," 19.90-91.

damage, wind stroke, and headache.[152] Ovate atractylodes was indicated for wind coldness, damp paralysis, dead flesh, and spastic jaundice.[153] The soybeans used medicinally were black soybeans, also called black beans, and were said to treat wind convulsions, wind paralysis, clenched mouth, and so on. Usually, the medical texts advised to heat-fry them, then immerse them in liquor to make a purple soybean decoction to be ingested by new mothers.[154] Ledebouriella, as its Chinese name *fangfeng* 防風 suggested, was indicated for all types of aversion to wind and wind evil.[155] Xu Zhicai from the Northern Qi said that "it cures women with wind in the uterus."[156] In addition to herbal medicines, methods of heating and massaging the soles of the feet and abdomen also expressed the idea that

[152] See recipes of *Jingui yaolüe*, 21.313; recipes of *Sengshenfang* and *Chanjing*, cited in *Ishinpo*, 23.34b; also cited in *Waitai miyao*, 34.953a. Also see *Qianjinfang*, 3.40-43. Regarding pueraria, the *Bielu* stated: "It grows in the mountain valleys of Wenshan 汶山." Tao Hongjing stated: "The best comes from the region between Nankang 南康 and Luling 廬陵." Su Song stated: "It is now available everywhere, but especially in Jiangsu and Zhejiang." See *Bencao gangmu*, "Herbs," 15.33-35.

[153] See recipes of *Xiaopinfang* and *Boji anzhongfang*, cited in *Waitai miyao*, 34.958ab. Also see *Chanjing*, cited in *Ishinpo*, 23.32a; and *Qianjinfang*, 3.40-43. The *Bielu* stated: "Ovate atractylodes grows in the valleys of Zhengshan 鄭山 and in Nanzheng 南鄭 of Hanzhong 漢中." Tao Hongjing stated: "Now it is available everywhere. The best is from Jiangshan 蔣山, Baishan 白山, and Maoshan 茅山." See *Bencao gangmu*, "Herbs," 11.4.

[154] See recipes of *Xiaopinfang* and *Luyanfang*, cited in *Ishinpo*, 23.31b-32b. Also see recipes of *Qianjinfang*, 3.40-43. The *Bielu* states: "Soybeans grow in level marshes on Taishan 泰山." Su Song stated: "It is now available everywhere." See *Bencao gangmu*, "Grains," 24.89-93.

[155] See *Jingui yaolüe*, 21.313; *Chanjing*, cited in *Ishinpo*, 23.34a; *Qianjinfang*, 3.40,42; and *Boji anzhongfang*, cited in *Waitai miyao*, 34.958ab. The *Bielu* states: "Ledebouriella grows in the streams and marshes of Shayuan 沙苑, as well as in Handan 邯鄲 [modern Hebei], Langya 瑯琊 [modern Anwei], and Shangcai 上蔡 [modern Henan]." Tao Hongjing stated: "Now the best comes from Pengcheng and Lanling 蘭陵 which are near Langya. It is also available from Baishi 百市 in Yuzhou 鬱州. The next best one comes from the border of Xiangyang 襄陽 and Yiyang 義陽." Su Gong stated: "Now the highest quality comes from Longshan 龍山 in Qizhou 齊州, but that from Zizhou 淄州, Yanzhou 兗州, or Qingzhou 青州 is also excellent." Su Song stated: "Now it is available in all the prefectures of east of Bian 汴, Huai 淮, and Zhe 浙." For all quotations, see *Bencao gangmu*, "Herbs," 11.47-49.

[156] See *Bencao gangmu*, "Herbs," 11.47-48. The same page also quotes Zhen Quan from the Northern Zhou who said that ledebouriella flowers treated "locking spasms of the four limbs, inability to walk, depletion and consumption of the channels, pain between the bones and joints, pain in the heart and abdomen." Su Gong from the Tang stated that ledebouriella seeds "are truly excellent for treating Wind."

"wind-stroke and contracting cold" was seen as the primary cause of convulsion illness.

The medical texts of early imperial China referred vaguely to the time when convulsion sickness erupted as "after birth," or "in childbed," or "in the hundred days postpartum."[157] But what exactly was meant when they discussed "convulsions" and "childbed wind"? Modern Chinese gynecological medicine assumes that it might have been weakness and depletion of *yin* and blood, catching a cold, or maybe infection and tetanus from childbirth-related injuries.[158] In the case of tetanus, given the level of medical practice at the time, it is very likely that the woman died within several days after giving birth; tetanus would not have lingered until a hundred days postpartum. If she suffered from weakness and depletion and contracted cold, then replenishment and preventing wind would indeed be important measures.

In fact, "contracting Wind evil" was a central concept in the medical literature for understanding postpartum illnesses. *Bingyuanlun*, volume forty-three, entitled "Symptoms of women's various postpartum illnesses," explained most illness symptoms as caused by "catching cold due to exposure to Wind," "long-term presence of Wind cold," or "being seized by Wind evil." Moreover, it claimed, if cold and cool evil *qi* flows into and stagnates in the waist and flanks, "in the case of subsequent pregnancies, miscarriage is likely," and it would influence her ability to reproduce afterwards.[159] For this reason, the medical care for the parturient woman did not end with the emergencies in the several days following delivery. The *Qianjinfang* used different expressions to designate the postpartum period, such as "new from birth" *xinchan* 新產, "just out of birth" *chuchan* 初產, "in the lying-in period" *ruzhong* 蓐中, "in childbed" *zairu* 在蓐, and "coming out of the lying-in period" *churu* 出蓐, and marked the seventh day as the starting point for nutrimental care:

> Within the first seven days postpartum, the evil blood is not yet exhausted and she may not ingest decoctions... after three or two days when the [lochia] is dispersed, she may take lycopodium pills. It is good to use the pills up within the [postpartum] month... In all cases, during the lying in period, she must

[157] See recipes of *Xiaopinfang*, cited in *Ishinpo*, 23.32a-33a; *Waitai miyao*, 34.953; and *Qianjinfang*, 3.40-43.
[158] See Luo Yuankai, *Zhongyi fukexue*, Ch. 10, "Postpartum illnesses."
[159] *Bingyuanlun*, 43.9.

> take lycopodium pills to replenish herself. The rule to use the [pills] is to take them after the [first] seven days and not any earlier.[160]

Considering the above-mentioned expression "three days of life and death" in the *Xiaopinfang* and the rule in the Song dynasty to lie in bed for three days, it seems that the first three days postpartum were a watershed for threats to a parturient woman's life. The period from the third to the seventh day was one of observation. If her condition did not turn into a life-threatening illness, then one could begin attending her with supplementing nutrients.

b) *Protecting Health in Childbed*

Protecting the mental and physical health of the new mother was definitely a central focus of concern in the medical texts. They recorded medical recipes for the treatment of all sorts of postpartum disorders, such as lochiorrhea, abnormal defecation and urination, heart and abdominal pain, agalactia, galactostasis, galactorrhea, prolapse, swelling, pain, and itching of the genitals as well as various kinds of depletion damages. With the exception of breast problems and vaginal pain, which were mostly managed with applications, baths, and similar methods, the majority of postpartum illnesses were treated with ingested medicinal prescriptions. Most supplementing medicinal decoctions from the seventh century on contained various kinds of meat.

For milk congestion (galactostasis) and overflow (galactorrhea), the medical texts suggested pressing heated stones on the breasts, covering the breasts with vinegar, applying a cooling rub of egg whites and lentils, or bathing then massaging the breasts with medicinal powders.[161] Vaginal prolapse with swelling and pain was mostly handled with heat treatments. They used iron flakes, tortoise blood, heated rat detritus, cnidium seeds, or peach kernel powder to hot-press or rub onto the genital area, or made decoctions with sulphur, medlar, peach leaves, and angelica to bathe the genital area or insert

[160] *Qianjinfang*, 3.36. For different expressions and terms for postpartum, see *Qianjinfang*, 3.36-50. Also see recipes of *Guangjifang*, *Jioujifang*, and *Xujenze chanhoufang* cited in *Waitai miyao*, 34.948ab, 958b. According to Ma Jixing, Xu Jenze practiced medicine and composed his medical works in the Tang dynasty.

[161] See recipes of *Geshifang*, cited in *Ishinpo*, 23.39b-40a; *Xiaopinfang*, cited in Tang Wanchun, *Xiaopinfang jilu jianzhu*, 122; *Jiyanfang*, cited in *Waitai miyao*, 34.943a-44a.

into the vagina as suppositories.[162] To treat the various postpartum illnesses by supplementing deficiency and nourishing the body, the most frequently chosen herbs were still licorice, fresh ginger, angelica, rehmannia, and cinnamon bark. Besides these, ginseng and peony were often on the list. Ginseng was considered to "supplement the five organs" and to "treat all deficiency syndromes."[163] Peony was said by medical texts to "free and disinhibit the flow of blood and *qi*," "treat Wind and replenish exhaustion," "cure all illnesses of women and all ailments before pregnancy and after birth."[164]

Tonification with meat varied depending on the time period and social status. The custom of congratulating a successful birth with sheep and liquor existed from the Han dynasty on. History recorded that Lu Wan 盧綰 (256- ? BCE) was born on the same day as Liu Bang 劉邦 (256-195 BCE), the founding emperor of the Han, and "the people of the village brought sheep and liquor to congratulate the two families."[165] Chen Yanzhi of the fifth century said that since childbirth was like awaiting death on the ground, as soon as it was completed, relatives would bring pig liver to celebrate.[166] In addition to mutton, the medicinal decoctions for replenishing deficiencies described in Tang medical texts like the *Qianjinfang* also contained deer meat, elk meat, roe deer meat, roe deer bones, and other delicacies, reflecting clearly that they were meant for elite households since they were not easy to obtain for the common people.[167]

---

[162] See recipes of *Xiaopinfang*, *Chanjing*, and *Jiyanfang*, cited in *Ishinpo*, 23.41a-42a; *Jiyanfang*, *Gujin luyanfang* 古今錄驗方, cited in *Waitai miyao*, 34.959b; *Qianjinfang*, 3.52-53.

[163] On ginseng, the *Bielu* states: "Ginseng grows in the mountain valleys of Shangdang 上黨 as well as in Liaodong 遼東." Su Gong said: "The most commonly used ginseng is the one from Korea Baiqi 百濟." Su Song stated: "Now it is available in all prefectures of east of the Yellow River and in Mount Tai, and there is also ginseng coming from Hebei Quechang 榷場 and central Fujiang, called Xinluo ginseng 新羅人參, but none of them are as excellent as the one from Shangdang." See *Bencao gangmu*, "Herbs," 12.88-96.

[164] On peony, the *Bielu* stated: "Peony grows in the river valleys and foothills of Zhongyue 中岳 [i.e., Songshan 嵩山]." Tao Hongjing stated: "Now the best comes from Baishan, Jiangshan, and Maoshan." Su Song stated: "Now it is available everywhere. The one from south of the Huai River is most excellent." See *Bencao gangmu*, "Herbs," 12.14-17.

[165] Sima Qian 司馬遷 (145-86 BCE), *Shiji* 史記 (Beijing: Zhonghua shuju, 1959), 93.2637.

[166] Cited in *Ishinpo*, 23.25a.

[167] *Qianjinfang*, 3.36-39. Also see *Cuishi*, cited in *Waitai miyao*, 34.943a.

In addition to the ingestion of medical decoctions, women in childbed were also expected to adjust their activities in order to heal their injuries and supplement their bodies. "wind stroke and contracting cold" was the primary explanation given in traditional medical texts for all postpartum illnesses, and the activities of the new mother were restricted in order to avoid wind. In ancient times when the privy was located outdoors, in order to prevent contracting wind, the lying-in woman "is particularly warned against going to the privy. It is better that she uses a bowl inside the room."[168] Sun Simiao suggested that engaging in sexual intercourse too early would cause women to suffer from "back problems of the wind *qi*, and depleting cold below the navel." Therefore he advised, "only a hundred days after birth may she engage in intercourse," and referred to the illness syndrome of a backward-arched body that was caused by not observing the prohibition against sexual intercourse as "childbed wind."[169]

The *Xiaopinfang* also mentions the idea that a woman should not engage in intercourse during the period of recovery, but explained it with the rationale that the woman's body had suffered injuries during delivery and needs time to recuperate:

> When a woman gives birth, the bones separate and open up in order to open the birth canal, and only then can the child come out. She will completely recover only after a hundred days are fulfilled. Women themselves are unaware of this and say that they have recovered to normal after merely fulfilling the month, [then] they have sexual intercourse and their activities damage the hundred channels. This then constitutes the diseases of the Five Taxations and Seven Damages, *wulao qishang* 五勞七傷.[170]

Although Chen Yanzhi did not yet regard sexual intercourse as the reason for contracting Wind, still, like Sun Simiao, he asked lying-in women to rest for about a hundred days. Obstetricians and gynecologists of the Song felt that sexual activity could influence the quality of the breast milk and therefore requested that women not engage in sexual intercourse when nursing. The *Chanjing* also mentioned that if a wet-nurse "nurses a child when panting from sexual intercourse ... it can kill the child. One must pay attention to this!"[171] But the words of Chen Yanzhi and Sun Simiao seemed

---

168 *Qianjinfang*, 3.36.
169 *Qianjinfang*, 3.36.
170 *Ishinpo*, 23.25ab.
171 *Ishinpo*, 25.8b.

to show that the taboo on sexual activity focused on the health of the new mother, rather than being an issue related to nursing.[172]

From the perspective of health preservation, most tonifying and replenishing prescriptions such as lycopodium pills might have been discontinued after fulfilling the month. If the new mother was not in good health, she needed continuous care and nourishment. The *Bingyuanlun* says that childbirth causes damage to the blood and *qi*. "When it is minor, care for and attend to her in moderation and she will achieve recovery within the month. When it is serious, even after the days of the month are completed, her *qi* and blood will still not be harmonious."[173] From the perspective of customs and taboos, fulfilling the month was indeed an important dividing line. *Xiaopinfang* said:

> The reason for a woman to fulfill the month after childbirth is because during the birth her body passes through a state of pollution. Before her lochia is cleansed, she is not allowed to go outdoors, neither to approach the locations of wells and stoves, nor to worship the spirits and attend ancestral sacrifices. Fulfilling the month does not mean to count until thirty days are full, but to step over one month. If one gives birth in the first month, stepping over the month means stepping over the second month and entering the third.[174]

This shows that a woman in childbed had to remain inside the delivery room for more than thirty days after delivery, whether for reasons of preserving her health or observing taboos, and only resumed her ordinary life after she had fulfilled the month. The entire task of childbirth, lasting from entering the month to this point, was finally concluded.

---

[172] *Ishinpo*, 25.8b, quoting the *Chanjing*. Both Sun Simiao, *Qianjinfang*, 5.74, and Wang Tao, *Waitai miyao*, 35.980, mentioned "methods to choose a wet nurse," which consider her features, personality, and health. But because "suitable appearances for a wet nurse include a great number of signs and one cannot ask for perfection," it is relatively brief, not like the complex and comprehensive demands of later medical literature and customs. On the employment of wet nurses in early imperial China, see Jen-der Lee, "Wet Nurses in Early Imperial China," *Nan Nü: Men, Women and Gender in Early and Imperial China* 2.1 (2000): 1-39. On their employment in the late imperial period, see Ping-chen Hsiung, "To Nurse the Young: Breastfeeding and Infant Feeding in Late Imperial China."

[173] *Bingyuanlun*, 43.11.

[174] *Ishinpo*, 23.25a.

The Social Meanings of Childbirth

Given the amount of suffering that the process of childbirth entailed, it is no wonder that it was considered a matter of life and death for women. However, while it certainly could mean a woman's survival or decease, the ramifications of its outcome went far beyond the woman's physical body. Perspectives on the birth by the parturient woman, the child, the husband, assistants, and doctors were sometimes identical, sometimes different; sometimes they coincided, sometimes they clashed. During the progression of birth, different types of interactions occurred, and in the end everybody enjoyed the rewards or shouldered the responsibility for the outcome together. The delivery as such was concluded when the fetus was born and the placenta had emerged, but the birth was not completely finished yet, and some time was required for the relationship between the mother and the surrounding society to be restored. This touches on questions of family relationships in a patriarchal society, the social status of the household, the criticism voiced by doctors against the birth attendants, and the images of women in childbirth. Based on information compiled from official histories, informal notes, and other sources, I will discuss the social meanings of childbirth in early imperial China under four topics.

a) *The Mother, her Baby, and its Father during Delivery*

In the ten months of pregnancy, the fetus was formed and nourished by the mother's body as if they were a single unit. When the days were fulfilled and the delivery due, the two had to separate. All of a sudden, the fetus was like an enemy in the mother's body, to the extent that the placenta and other substances on which the child's survival had depended could endanger the mother's life.[175] A so-called smooth birth referred to the smooth progression of separation, which might otherwise jeopardize the safety of both mother and child. The process of delivery influenced the feelings of mother and child, especially in the case of a breech or other adverse positions. The *Zuozhuan* 左傳 stated that, in the first year of Duke of Yin, "the Duke of Zhuang was born adversely, alarming [his mother] Lady

[175] For the relations between placenta, fetus, and mother, see Li Jianmin, "Mawangdui Hanmu boshu 'Yuzang maibaotu' jianzheng."

Jiang 姜, therefore she named him *Wusheng* 寤生 (adversely born) and detested him." One version of the meaning of *wusheng* was the feet emerging before the head.[176] In the Han, this was greatly abhorred and was one reason among the people to abandon a child.[177]

The extant information is insufficient to judge whether the experience of birth influenced the future attitude of the child towards his or her parents. The mother of Fan Ye 范曄, author of the dynastic history of the Later Han, delivered him while in the privy. She was unable to catch him in time with her hands, and Fan Ye's forehead was injured on the bricks. The biography of Fan Ye in the *Songshu* recorded that when Ye broke the law and was about to be punished, his mother struck him on the neck and cheek and said, crying, "You do not consider my old age. What shall I do this day?" and Ye "did not show the slightest remorse." After the execution, the court took over Fan Ye's household and found his concubines dressed up ornately while his mother lived in poverty, having only one cook to help with the firewood." [178] Unfortunately, there is not enough information to judge whether Ye's unfilial behavior was related to the circumstances of his birth, but this kind of historical research into psychology should be quite fascinating.

Based on the medical literature of early imperial China, it is impossible to answer unequivocally the question of who led the process of delivery. Both the *Zhuyue yangtaifang* and *Qianjinfang* which included it stated that, "when the days are fulfilled, the birth will come," and "await the time, and the birth will come." Therefore, at the very least, doctors did not consider that the pregnant woman had any way to influence the beginning or the end of delivery. The surviving medical sources did not offer enough case studies to determine whether abdominal pain was ultimately a result of the uterus trying to expel the fetus and therefore contracting, or of the fetus stretching outwards because it was unable to stay in the uterus any longer.[179] Medicinal prescriptions for treating a dead fetus in

---

[176] For Duke Zhuang's story, see Yang Bojun 楊伯峻, *Chunqiu zuozhuanzhu* 春秋左傳注, 10. In addition to the definition "adversely born," Ying Shao 應劭 (32-92) also explained *wusheng* as "born with open eyes." See Ying Shao, *Fengsu tongyi* 風俗通義, annotated by Wang Liqi 王利器 (Beijing: Zhonghua shuju, 1981), hereafter cited as *Fengsu tongyi jiaozhu* 風俗通義校注.

[177] Li Zhende, "Han Sui zhijian de 'shengzi buju' wenti," 752.

[178] *Songshu*, 69.1828-29.

[179] Research on the history of Western obstetrics indicates that doctors from

the abdomen and a retained placenta were identical in many places, indicating that doctors recognized uterine contractions to be an important driving force during delivery. The methods of getting on the ground and squatting on straw as well as sitting and lying according to her wishes also suggested that the parturient woman could assist herself during delivery.[180] However, in many other situations, the fetus was seen as the main driving force in delivery. The mother's safety was mostly determined by its movement towards the vagina. In the case of breech or other adverse presentations, doctors worried that "the child will rise up to press against the heart" and employed all sorts of methods like scratching with fingernails or poking with needles to make the child turn back around by itself. In particular, they believed that writing the father's name on the fetus's sole would cause the child to emerge smoothly.[181] They also suggested that if the mother swallowed a pill made of the husband's pubic hair and cinnabar paste, the "child would emerge holding the pill in its hand."[182] Apparently, they believed that the fetus was able to recognize its own father.

The idea that the fetus was able to discern its father indirectly showed the importance of the husband during delivery. Because of the idea of childbirth impurity since ancient times and the tradition that husbands were barred from the delivery room in the modern era, the husband has often been depicted as merely pacing nervously outside the room. However, the various measures employed to treat childbirth complications in early imperial period indicated that, at least among the common people, the woman's husband, being the

---

ancient to medieval times believed that delivery was directed by the fetus who had matured and wanted to leave the mother's abdomen. See Gélis, *History of Childbirth*, 141.

180 In modern childbirth, women mostly enter the hospital and give birth in the supine position, being directed by medical personnel in the process. The popularity of Caesarean sections even introduces the possibility of delivering unconsciously without the cooperation of the mother. In comparison, the independent style of childbirth in ancient society expresses the active role of women in the process of birth. The changes in childbirth assistance and the control of women by institutionalized medicine are important topics in the history of Western medicine and women's history. See Shorter, *A History of Women's Bodies*, 56-57; Odent, *Birth Reborn*; and Gélis, *History of Childbirth*, 121-33. However, in the context of Chinese history, related issues were raised only in the recent past.

181 Recipe of *Jiyanfang*, cited in *Ishinpo*, 23.13b.

182 Recipe of *Jiyanfang*, cited in *Waitai miyao*, 33.934b.

fetus's father, could have played an important role. In rural nuclear families, the husband might have been needed to assist the woman at the onset of her labor pains to spread out the grass and arrange things properly, as well as finding other people for support and relief. While waiting for female relatives, friends, neighbors, or the midwife to arrive, if he was indeed not inside the delivery room, he must have surely waited nearby to offer help in case of an emergency. In some circumstances, he might have to enter the delivery room several times in order to solve complications by "spitting water into the woman's mouth."[183] However, when it was difficult to save both mother and child, whether the woman or her husband would make the final decision may have differed depending on the situation.

The *Qidong yeyu* 齊東野語 (Wild talk from the eastern Qi) recorded a childbirth story of the Tang:

> Empress Zhangsun 長孫 of the Tang was pregnant with [the future] Emperor Gao 高宗. When the birth was pending, she was unable to deliver for several days. Imperial doctor Li Dongxuan 李洞玄 was summoned to diagnose her pulse and reported to the Empress, "Because the child's hand is clutching the mother's heart, it cannot be born." Emperor Tai 太宗 asked, "What could be done?" Li Dongxuan said, "If the child is saved, the mother will not survive; if the mother survives, the child must die." The Empress said, "Save the child, and the empire will enjoy eternal fortune" ... Subsequently, [Li Dongxuan] lanced through her abdomen with a needle, penetrating to the heart until it reached the [child's] hand. The Empress perished, and the heir-apparent was born. Later when the weather was cloudy, his [the heir-apparent's] hand would show scars. ... Pang Anchang 龐安常 who watched for complications in pregnant women said, "Although the child has already emerged from the uterus, it clutches in its hands the mother's intestines or stomach, and it will not let go of the placenta. Find the hand of the child and needle it on the *hukou* 虎口 [between the thumb and the index finger], [so] the child will draw back its hand and be born again. [Then] take a look at the *hukou*, and you will see the scars."[184]

---

[183] Recipe of *Jiyanfang*, cited in *Ishinpo*, 23.13b; and *Waitai miyao*, 33.934a. See Figure 3 for a vivid depiction of childbirth. The man on the scene is better understood as the husband of the laboring woman than an overseeing male doctor, since the theme of this twelfth-century sculpture is the unrepayable love of one's parents. Studying the history of childbirth in rural France, Gélis points out that the husband, because of his physical strength, was sometimes responsible for holding up the laboring woman at the waist and for carrying her back to the bed. But since the husband mostly entered the picture in the case of childbirth complications, his appearance was, from the perspective of the parturient woman, also a sign of danger and cause for alarm. See Gélis, *History of Childbirth*, 101-3.

[184] Zhou Mi 周密 (1232-98), *Qidong yeyu*, in *Tang Song shiliao biji congkan* 唐宋史料筆記叢刊 (Beijing: Zhonghua shuju, 1983), 14.250-52.

On the one hand, these stories illustrate the influence of the fetus in delivery, but on the other, they illuminate the power relations between the wife, the fetus, and the husband in a patriarchal society. Empress Zhangsun's decision to sacrifice her life for the sake of the empire seemed to show that women also considered themselves to be merely a birthing tool for continuing the patriarchal line. Nevertheless, in most situations of childbirth complications, the woman might have lost consciousness and therefore been unable to express an opinion, leaving the husband to be the one making the final decision. Regarding this issue, there is practically no historical information for discussion. However, the common people in the early imperial period should not be put in the same light with the Tang imperial family or officials' households. In the nuclear family of the commoners, the main wife was the most important source of labor; even though the patriarchal family may have yearned for offspring, it may not have chosen to preserve the child over the mother's life. Otherwise the common people would not have practiced infant abandonment in cases of adverse births.[185]

b) *Differences in Medical Care between the Rich and the Poor*

Many questions can be raised by the hypothesis that social status created differences in childbirth, but useful historical sources are few. Based on his own observations, the doctor cited in *Waitai miyao* claimed a difference in social status, stating that "poor maidservants giving birth alone" did not have complications, and that "most deaths in childbirth occur in elite families." While there may be some merit in this statement, it cannot cover all aspects of the subject.

First, the resources that families were able to provide for the woman in her final stage of pregnancy differed greatly. Among the general population, most households in early imperial China were nuclear families in which the wife constituted an important source of labor. It was impossible for her to rest from her work because of pregnancy, and she most likely continued to toil until right be-

[185] For reasons for infanticide and child abandonment, see Li Zhende, "Han-Sui zhijian de 'shengzi buju' wenti." For the role and status of women in the context of begetting a son for the patriarchal family in early imperial China, see Li Zhende (Jender Lee), "Han-Tang zhijian qiuzi yifang shitan: jianlun fuke lanshang yu xingbie lunshu" 漢唐之間求子醫方試探—兼論婦科濫觴與性別論述 *Bulletin of the Institute of History and Philology, Academia Sinica* 68.2 (1997): 283-367.

fore delivery. In the literati class, stem families and extended families were increasing in this period. With relatives and friends in addition to servants in the household, more human resources were available, which may have allowed the woman a chance to rest in the last stage of pregnancy.[186] As for preparations when entering the month, elite families were probably able to set up a tent or construct a hut according to the birth charts, but the complexity of preparations most likely decreased progressively with the extent of poverty among the ordinary people. History records that "Gou Jian 句踐 was assigned a position in the Wu 吳 and his wife followed him. Along the way, she gave birth to a daughter in a depot." Also, Cao Cao's 曹操 Queen Bian卞, who came from a prostitute's family, was born in a "white depot of the Qi district."[187] Apparently, pregnant women did not receive special care simply because of an impending delivery. The *Soushenji* 搜神記 (Records of searching for spirits) also recorded a story in which a very poor woman worked right up to the birth and "delivered her child in the wilderness while gathering firewood."[188]

Secondly, between the Sui and the Tang dynasties, doctors had a more systematic view regarding the progression of labor, necessary time, and number of assistants. Elite families might have been exposed to and accepted new ideas regarding delivery somewhat earlier than the common people. While the cultivation of medicinal herbs, whether for making the fetus slippery or for treating childbirth complications, increased gradually, herbs that were grown in specific areas were probably obtained more easily by elite families than by the common people. And when it came to caring for the new mother, they were also able to provide more tonifying, replenishing, and nutritious foods.

However, there must have been some knowledge regarding the topic of childbirth that was shared by all, whether rich or poor, such

---

[186] For detailed discussions of the size and composition of households in early imperial China, see Tang Changru 唐長孺, "Menfa de xingcheng jiqi shuailuo" 門閥的形成及其衰落, in *Wuhan daxue renwen kexue xuebao* 武漢大學人文科學學報 8 (1959), 1-24; Xu Zhuoyun (Cho-yun Hsü) 許倬雲, *Handai jiating daxiao* 漢代家庭大小, in Xu, *Qiugubian* 求古編 (Taipei: Lianjing chubanshe, 1982), 515-41; Du Zhengsheng (Cheng-sheng Tu) 杜正勝, "Lizhi, jiaozu yu lunli" 禮制, 家族與倫理, in Du, *Gudai shehui yu guojia* 古代社會與國家 (Taipei: Yunchen wenhua chubanshe, 1992), 729-876.

[187] *Yuejueshu* 越絕書, cited in *Taiping yulan*, 194.9b; *Sanguozhi*, 5.156.

[188] *Taiping yulan*, 362.9b-10a.

as the concept of the mutual influence of Heaven and the human realm, and the correspondence of all things, as well as the idea that "great speed and little pain constitute a smooth birth." As for noisy environment, while the common people might not have many surrounding relatives to observe the delivery, it is still very likely that neighbors and friends would come to help. Among the various recipes for treating complications, many advised getting "chicken eggs from three households," "salt from three households," and "water from three households" as well as "rice from three households" in order to make a medicinal prescription that was aimed at inducing a smooth birth.[189] This shows that delivery could be an affair that the whole village participated in. Substances from the neighbors' households were believed to resolve complications in birth and, even if the neighbors did not enter the delivery room itself, they still could create hubbub by going in and out of the laboring woman's house. It was not like the statement in *Waitai miyao*, "poor maidservants giving birth alone."

Lastly, if complications did occur, all households probably administered a variety of treatments in combination and, in their search for quick results, placed their faith both in shamans and in medicine regardless of social status. The Jin dynasty story of Yu Fakai 于法開 (ca. fourth century) who used needling to treat a childbirth complication illustrated the chaotic situation when "the entire range of treatments were ineffective and the whole family was frantic."

> In the Jin dynasty, Yu Fakai of Mt. Yanbai 剡白 was a man of unknown origin. He served Master Lan 蘭 as his disciple. He sat alone in deep contemplation, and his words showed distinctive insight. He was learned in the Fangguang Sutra 放光經 and Lotus Sutra. Moreover, he continued [to study] *Qipo* (耆婆, Jivaka in Sanskrit) and was well versed in medicine. Once, when he was begging for food and came to a master's house, the woman who was giving birth was in great danger, and the entire range of treatments was ineffective, so the whole family was frantic. Kai said: "This is easy to treat." Just then, the master was about to slaughter a goat to make a sacrifice to unauthorized deities. Kai first took a little meat to make broth, asked the woman to drink it completely, and then he followed the *qi* and needled her. In an instant, the child emerged with the amnion enclosing it.[190]

---

[189] For instance, see *Jiyangfang* cited in *Waitai miyao*, 33.935; and *Chanjing* cited in *Ishinpo*, 23.14.

[190] Hui Jiao 慧皎 (497-554), *Gaosengzhuan*, annotated by Tang Yongtong 湯用彤 (Beijing: Zhonghua shuju, 1992), 4.167-68.

This story from the *Gaosengzhuan* 高僧傳 (Biographies of eminent monks) was recorded to propagate Buddhism and therefore expressed the connection between Buddhist monks and medicine, representing rationality, which was in contrast with the unauthorized sacrifices, representing superstition. The description of the child emerging after the mother was needled clearly showed the efficacy of poking with a needle to induce childbirth, identical to stories about Hua Tuo 華陀 in the third century and Xu Wenbo 徐文伯 in the fifth.[191] Nevertheless, poking with a needle belonged to the category of distinguished skills which average households would have hardly been able to take advantage of. Although the text did not specify what was included under the "entire range of treatments that were ineffective," it is most likely that for the laboring woman's safety, all the various methods were used in combination, resulting in the simultaneous resort to medicine and magic. But it is quite doubtful that a male doctor would be invited to visit the scene unless it was a case of birth complications.

c) *The Development of Gynecology and Obstetrics and the Issue of Midwifery*

In ancient times, pregnant women probably did not have regular prenatal examinations. The famous doctor Hua Tuo from the third century was reported to have examined the pregnant wives of eminent officials and found fetuses having died in the abdomen. When a high official's wife suffered from abdominal pain and unrest in the sixth month of pregnancy, Hua Tuo observed her pulse and said, "The fetus is already dead."[192] When Hua Tuo was called in to observe a general's ill wife, he found that "the dead fetus is

---

[191] Hua Tuo used the needle to make a dead fetus descend; see *Sanguozhi*, 29.799. Xu Wenbo induced a birth by acupuncture; see Li Yanshou (ca. seventh century), *Nanshi* 南史 (Beijing: Zhonghua shuju, 1975), 32.838. For needling to induce birth, see Li Zhende, "Han-Sui zhijian de 'shengzi buju' wenti," 787-95. The above-mentioned Zhou Mi from the Song dynasty in his *Qidong yeyu*, 14.250-52 "Needling and Lancing," recorded the needling methods of Li Dongxuan and Pang Anchang, both penetrating the mother's abdomen to place the needle directly into the child's hand. This was different from the above-mentioned treatment for breech or adverse presentation in the *Xiaopinfang* in which the fetus was poked with a needle in order to make it recoil and turn around, which again differed from the method of poking the mother with a needle to induce delivery, used by Hua Tuo, Xu Wenbo, Yu Fakai, and others.

[192] *Sanguozhi*, 29.799.

withered and parched, and the circumstances are so that it will not be delivered by itself." Therefore, in order to make it descend, Hua Tuo needled the mother and made her ingest tonics.[193] Although these two ladies did summon a doctor during pregnancy to examine them, in both cases it was because they were of ill health. It is difficult to determine whether they would have necessarily undergone a medical examination at a certain period, even in the case of elite wives, if they had not encountered problems in their pregnancies.[194] If no complications were anticipated, a doctor was not necessarily summoned even when delivery was impending. The *Bingyuanlun* stated repeatedly how the attendants should have held up a woman's waist and what the birth helpers should have done, proving that the most important people to assist in delivery were indeed not the doctor. Nevertheless, doctors did have opinions regarding a normal delivery and also held on to the idea that birth assistants may have lost control and created deadly risks for the parturient woman.

In the development of gynecology and obstetrics in China, the seventh century witnessed a theoretical breakthrough. The fact that

[193] *Hou Hanshu*, 82.2738.

[194] Women's medical treatment in ancient times is quite difficult to determine. But from a few sources we know that in early imperial China it might not have been prohibited for women to consult a male doctor and be examined. In the ninth volume of Wang Shuhe's *Maijing*, several entries began with the phrase "a woman came to be examined." These women most likely came from the upper class. Wang Shuhe referred to them as "ladies," or described how "a well-dressed woman came for an examination." Among these, one entry also illustrates the situation of a mother bringing her daughter to receive medical treatment. The record goes as follow.

> A woman brings in a girl of fifteen years old for examination. The woman says that the girl menstruated at the age fourteen, but now her menstruation has stopped. The mother expresses her fear. The master asks, "Is this girl your own daughter? If she is, I will tell you the reason." The woman answers, "Of course she is my daughter." The master says, "The reason I am asking is no other than that you yourself also began menstruating at the age of fourteen. Therefore I diagnose this as the [medical condition of] *binian* 避年 [lit. "skipping a year," i.e., menstrual irregularity in which menstruation stops for a year after the first time]. Do not think it strange; later it should naturally resume its flow." *Maijing*, 9.8b.

From this, we can see that the mother had herself come for an examination when she was fourteen and now also took her daughter when she was fifteen, similar to the practice of going to a "family doctor." Also, the fact that the doctor remembered the mother's symptoms when she was fourteen could have reflected the doctor's memory, or it could mean that he kept a file of medical histories. There was a record of keeping medical cases in the *Zhouli* 周禮, and the Han doctor Chunyu Yi 淳于意 also compiled *zhenji* 診籍 [Registration of diagnoses]. It would not be surprising if Wang Shuhe kept an archive of special medical cases.

the *Bingyuanlun* placed the topics of menstruation, vaginal discharge, and other conditions before pregnancy and birth had an impact during later periods on establishing the categorization of gynecology and obstetrics into the sections of menstruation, vaginal discharge, pregnancy, and delivery.[195] And between the third and the seventh centuries, doctors' ideas about women and delivery also became progressively systematic. First, medicinal prescriptions for making the fetus slippery originally failed to identify the exact time of their use, but gradually the appropriate months for different types of decoctions were specified. Second, due to the efforts of doctors, the structure and content of the birth charts which had been separated into different categories and based on various theories were gradually unified under a set of standardized rules. Third, the time frame of postpartum medical care became increasingly specific in the medical literature, from the general expression "after birth" to the special characteristics of each period, from three days, seven days, fulfilling the month, to a hundred days. At the same time, the doctors also proposed explanations for childbirth complications besides breaking taboos and offending the spirits.[196] The *Bingyuanlun*, *Qianjinfang*, and *Waitai miyao* coincided in their criticism of the birth assistants. In the opinion of the doctors, their greatest fault lay in affecting the laboring woman's emotional state with their worrying and anxiety, and their tendency to hurry towards the completion of labor was sufficient to create childbirth complications.[197]

---

[195] Ma Dazheng, *Zhongguo fuchanke fazhanshi*, 90.

[196] Furth suggests that "fulfilling the month" and "one hundred days" are two perspectives from different contexts, the former emerging earlier and focusing on the impurity of birth in a ritualistic context, and the latter appearing somewhat later and focusing on nurturing and recuperating in a medical context. The most significant aspect of childbirth in terms of ritual was to avoid breaking taboos and offending the spirits. See Charlotte Furth, "Ming Qing Medicine and the Construction of Gender," *Jindai Zhongguo funüshi yanjiu* 近代中國婦女史研究 2 (1994): 229-50. The present article, indicating the vicissitudes and standardization of both aspects between the Sui and Tang, clearly shows that "fulfilling the month" also constituted an important stage for nourishing and tonifying the parturient woman in the medical context, rather than just marking the end point of ritual taboos.

[197] It is impossible to determine from the sources in the early imperial period whether the laboring woman might have spent her energy too early and the assistants intervened excessively because women were always expected to toil hard, including struggling without slacking during childbirth. Furth mentions this possibility in her research of delivery during the Qing dynasty. See Charlotte Furth, "Concepts of Pregnancy, Childbirth, and Infancy in Ch'ing China," *Journal of Asian Studies* 46.1 (1987): 7-55.

The doctors assumed that when a woman was in labor, her family, as well as assistants with insufficient experience, tended to try to shorten the time in order to complete the delivery as fast as possible, whereas the doctors advocated allowing the birth to follow its natural course. Chao Yuanfang, for example, urged the birth assistants to wait until the laboring woman felt pain both in her abdomen and waist before holding up her waist, and to tie the umbilical cord to something and wait for the placenta to descend naturally. Sun Simiao stressed that, at the time of delivery, there should be no more than two to three people attending. And Wang Tao, with his quotation of Cui Zhiti's text, apparently agreed that a woman was able to feel safe and self-possessed when giving birth alone, and that it was unnecessary to "gather women around her" since it led to inappropriate behavior.

In fact, while most of those who performed midwifery did not necessarily live on their skill, there were women since early times in China who worked as birth attendants for a living. Birth assistants might have helped out in other women's births because of their poverty and need for an income, or they might have been women with a lot of personal experience. Their fame as "being skilled at observing birth" gradually spread in the countryside, and the public regarded such people as midwives. Historical records mention that a certain Mu Yu's 木羽 mother from the Han dynasty "presided over birth assistance because of her poverty."[198] A marvel story from the fourth century told of the woman Su Yi 蘇易 who was so famous in the countryside for "being skilled at observing birth" that "a female tiger, about to give birth, was unable to deliver and, on the verge of death, kept staring at her. She realized [the tiger's intention], sought for [the fetus] and took it out."[199] At the delivery of imperial consorts, female doctors would have been summoned to help.[200] In the case of an average women, there was most probably no doctor present, and the woman was assisted by female relatives and friends with experience in childbirth. Su Yi's story shows that

198 *Taiping yulan*, vol. 361, quoting the *Liexianzhuan*.

199 Gan Bao, *Soushenji*, 20.237, entry on "Su Yi."

200 When Empress Xu 許 of Han Emperor Xuan (73-49 BCE) was approaching delivery, the female doctor Chunyu Yan 淳于衍 was summoned to enter the palace to help. For the story that Chunyu Yan was threatened and bribed by another consort's mother to kill Empress Xu with a poisonous pill made with aconite seeds, see *Hanshu*, 8.251, 97a.3966.

when complications did arise, villagers relied on the woman who had a reputation of "being skilled at observing birth."[201]

Since male doctors were for the most part summoned only in the case of complications and had in fact less experience of direct participation, it has always been a controversial issue in the history of gynecology and obstetrics whether or not their criticism of the aptitude of female birth assistants was justified. Midwives did not transmit written texts to record their skills and techniques for delivering babies and did not have their own voice in the history of gynecology and obstetrics. Maybe, therefore, one should interpret the fact that doctors blamed birth assistants for causing childbirth complications only as a kind of rhetoric.[202] In early imperial Chinese medical literature, the materia medica and tonifying decoctions used for prenatal

---

[201] Wang Tao cited from Cui Zhiti, recording a story of a man who "having had one older sister and two daughters all die in childbirth, therefore was greatly troubled and anxious when his pregnant daughter-in-law was approaching the month of delivery." The man went into the mountains to find a doctor who personally took charge of the delivery at his home. This should be seen as an exception. See *Waitai miyao*, 33.923-24.

[202] Discussions of this kind, or even debates, have already lasted for many years in the history of gynecology and obstetrics in the West, and midwifery and its history has become an important research topic. See Shorter, *A History of Women's Bodies*, the section on "A history of birth experience." Also see Ornella Moscucci, *The Science of Women: Gynaecology and Gender in England, 1800-1929* (Cambridge: Cambridge University Press, 1990). In the context of Chinese history, this subject has not been vigorously debated due to the scarcity of writings. Studies in medical history indicate that doctors in the Song attached themselves to the ranks of Confucian scholars, attempting to raise their social status. Moreover, gynecology and obstetrics became a specialized field in the Song, and it is not hard to imagine the competition between doctors and midwives. From the Yuan dynasty on, midwives fell into the category of the "three nuns and six grannies," who occupied a lower social standing. However, scholars have also pointed out that such categorization by the Confucian literati did not necessarily reflect people's experience with female doctors nor did it represent the reputation of midwives among male doctors. For the relationship between doctors and Confucians, see Chen Yuanpeng 陳元朋, "Songdai de ruyi: jianping Robert P. Hymes youguan Song-Yuan yizhe diwei de lundian" 宋代的儒醫—兼評 Robert P. Hymes 有關宋元醫者地位的論點, *Xinshixue* 新史學 6.1 (1995): 194-202. For the development of gynecology and obstetrics in the Song and the male doctors' relations with midwives, see Furth, *A Flourishing Yin*. For the social ramifications of categorizing some women as "three nuns and six grannies" and a general survey of female doctors and midwives in Chinese history, see Angela K. C. Leung, "Women Practicing Medicine in Pre-modern China," in Harriet Zurndorfer, ed., *Chinese Women in the Imperial Past: New Perspectives* (Leiden: Brill, 1999), 101-34. For discussion on women healers specifically in early imperial China, see Li Zhende (Jen-der Lee), "Han-Tang zhijian de nüxing yiliao zhaoguzhe," 漢唐之間的女性醫療照顧者, *Taida lishi xuebao* 台大歷史學報 23 (1999): 123-56.

preparation and postpartum recovery expanded progressively and became increasingly complex. But delivery still retained its unpredictable characteristics, and situations occurring on the birth scene invited different interpretations. With the outcome being difficult to foresee, the doctors' reprimanding the birth attendants might be understood as their intention to search for some new explanations in addition to traditional prohibitions and taboos.

In fact, doctors, households, and birth assistants were all deeply convinced that childbirth involved supernatural forces. As mentioned in the beginning of this article, both the Han dynasty imperial household and the common people worshipped Shenjun. Besides reflecting their fear of childbirth complications, this also revealed the belief that those who had died in childbirth had the ability to deliver other women from complications. In the early imperial period, on the one hand, doctors' records showed a systematic transformation of the birth charts, criticisms of birth assistants, and the introduction of new medicinal decoctions, leading the way to the medical management of childbirth. But on the other hand, by passing on practices of isolation and taboos, they also transmitted a childbirth culture that was identical to that of the common people.[203]

d) *Isolation, Taboos, and the Inauspicious Nature of Childbirth*

While delivery was the very core of childbirth, the birth did not begin or end there. From the perspective of the parturient woman herself as well as her relatives, friends, and neighbors, the process of birth was marked by isolation and taboos, from the time of entering the month and setting up the tent to fulfilling the month and coming out of the lying-in period. The isolation began with sending the woman off for the birth and setting up the hut. Before the delivery, she was forced to leave her regular daily life and enter a location that had been arranged specifically for her. The central idea behind her isolation was the inauspicious nature of childbirth.

Although the earliest surviving information regarding setting up the hut is found in the *Chanjing*, the practice of sending the woman off for the birth might have already existed in the Spring and Autumn period (722-481 BCE). The *Zuozhuan* recorded that "at the birth of

[203] That childbirth itself carried the weight of mystery and uncertainty is well illustrated in the belief of the "ghost fetus." See Yi-Li Wu, "Ghost Fetuses."

Gong Yan 公衍 and Gong Wei 公爲, both their mothers emerged." Du Yu's 杜預 (222-84) annotation of this was "they emerged from the *chanshe* 產舍 (delivery house)."[204] The fact that the two mothers together entered the delivery house, awaited childbirth, and afterwards came out together shows that women did not give birth in the space of their daily lives. The custom of sending a woman off to give birth in a delivery house, which also existed in the Han dynasty, is illustrated by two examples in Ying Shao's 應劭 *Fengsu tongyi* 風俗通義 (General explanations of customs), showing that inside the delivery house, the wife of a government official might have been lying next to the wife of a butcher:

> There was a rich family in Yingchuan 潁川, in which the older and younger brothers lived together. Their two wives were both pregnant and, after several months, the older wife injured her fetus and secluded herself to hide this. When the time of birth arrived, they went to the *rushe* 乳舍 [birth house] together. The younger brother's wife gave birth to a son and [the older brother's wife] stole it that night. They fought in court for three years, but the district prefect was unable to come to a decision.[205]

> Zhou Ba 周霸 of Runan 汝南, named Wengzhong 翁仲, was a clerk to the Defender-in-Chief (*taiweiyuan* 太尉掾). His wife gave birth to a daughter in the birth house and was greatly upset about not having a son. At that time, a butcher's wife lying next to her gave birth to a son, and she privately exchanged her own baby [for the butcher's son], giving [the butcher's wife] tens of thousands of money.[206]

---

[204] *Zuozhuan* 左傳, in *Shisanjing zhushuben*, 53.922. The annotation by Kong Yingda 孔穎達 (574-648) on the same page suggests that in Du Yu's commentary the "delivery house" was identical to the *ceshi* 側室 (side room) mentioned in the *Liji*. But the side room was a room that was already attached to the house, which was different from the birth house, used specifically for sending the mother off to give birth. If what Du Yu called "delivery house" was identical to the "birth house," then the Jin period in which Du Yu lived followed the same custom as the Han, sending the mother off to give birth in the delivery house, whereas Kong Yingda's explanation of the delivery house as the side room might show that the custom of sending the laboring women to the birth house had already been abandoned by the Tang.

[205] *Fengsu tongyi jiaozhu*, 590.

[206] *Fengsu tongyi jiaozhu*, 591. This story continued:

> Later, Wengzhong became minister of Beihai. His official Zhou Guang 周光 was able to see ghosts. He appointed him to become recorder and sent him to return to his home prefecture and province in order to sacrifice to the ancestors … Arriving at the top of the ancestral burial mound, the young gentleman [Wengzhong's son] sprinkled libations for the sacrifice while the recorder crouched low behind his back, but all he could see was a butcher with tattered clothes and a spiral-shaped headdress, squatting in front of the ancestral tablets, holding a knife and slicing off meat whereas there were several people dressed in green clothes and with their seals of office who went to and fro between the

The brothers from Yingchuan were from a rich household; they certainly should not have lacked a room to use or servants to employ during childbirth. The butcher's wife also went to the birth house, lying right next to the official's wife; thus the birth house did not constitute a special medical treatment reserved for the upper classes. Why would they go to a birth house for delivery?

Wang Chong 王充 (27-91) criticized the fact that in Jiangnan 江南, people "shun women in childbirth, considering it inauspicious, and in order to make it auspicious, [the woman] enters the mountains and forests, going far away, and crossing rivers and marshes, while nobody interacts with her. The family of the woman also avoids and abhors her. Graveyards, cottages, even roadsides she may enter only after having passed through the month, aversion to her is this great." But at the same time, he explained that the situation was not like that in Jiangbei 江北.[207] Both Yingchuan and Runan, the above-mentioned two examples, were located in the Jiangbei area.[208] These four women did not give birth at home but went to a birth house. Couldn't this mean that, although in the Jiangbei area where laboring women were not avoided and abhorred the way they were in Jiangnan, it was also customary to send them off to give birth elsewhere?[209]

> mausoleums of the east and west wings of the main building, not daring to come in ... Wengzhong asked his wife, "why do you raise this kid?"... the old woman was speechless and overcome by emotions, then in tears explained exactly the reason for this. At that time, their son was already eighteen. [Wengzhong] bid him farewell, saying, "Whenever one has sons, one wants them to continue the ancestral line, but if the ancestors are not enjoying the sacrifice, I am helpless."

Ying Shao stated in his summary: "The fact that the ancestors' ghosts do not accept sacrifices that are not from their kind is very clear. How can people adopt a son from another lineage?"

[207] Wang Chong, *Lunheng* 論衡, in *Xinbian zhuzi jicheng* 新編諸子集成 (Taipei: Shijie shuju, 1983), 228.

[208] Yingchuan was located in the Yu 禹 district of modern Henan, and Runan in the southeast of Shangcai and northeast of Pingyu 平輿 in modern Henan. For historical maps of the Han dynasty, see Tan Qixiang 譚其驤, ed., *Zhongguo lishi dituji* 中國歷史地圖集 (Shanghai: ditu chubanshe, 1982), vol. 2, 19-20.

[209] The custom of sending women off to give birth may not have ended with the Han. In the political upheaval in the early Jin dynasty, it was said that "a woman suddenly appeared at the door of the Commander-in-Chief, requesting to stay for her delivery," saying, "I will leave right after having cut the cord." See *Jinshu*, 29.907. During the tyrannical rule of Lord Donghun 東昏侯 (499-500) in the Southern Qi (479-502), the historians recorded that "families of married women in childbirth removed them for delivery and lodged them in another dwelling." See *Nan Qi Shu*,

Although a woman in childbirth was forced to leave the space of her daily life and was very likely to be sent off to a different place for delivery, people in the Han considered it inappropriate for a married woman to return to her natal family to give birth. The *Fengsu tongyi* explains: "It is not appropriate to return home for the birth. The custom has it that it leads to people's downfall. [Ying Shao's] comment: Because women like to take their daughters and exchange them for other people's sons, therefore do not permit them to return home."[210] From the comment, we can see that the idea of valuing sons more than daughters in childbirth might have caused women to exchange their own daughters for other people's sons, and the families of women in childbirth therefore took serious precautions to prevent that.[211] However, both Ying Shao and Wang Chong were known for using rationality to criticize the customs and beliefs of their contemporaries, and therefore might have searched for the rational explanation for the prohibition against allowing women to return home for the birth. From the perspective of popular sayings, it is clear that people's true worry was that returning home for birth might have caused the natal family to decline. Obviously this is similar to the custom in Jiangnan criticized by Wang Chong, also being rooted in the concept of the inauspiciousness of childbirth.

Even if women did not go to a delivery house or return to their natal home, from the Han dynasty on, it was customary to set up a

7.103. But the emphasis of the above story was on predicting that the King of Qi was about to be murdered, being that the pronunciation of the word for umbilical cord was also "*qi*" in Chinese. The story itself is probably insufficient in proving that the custom of sending women away for childbirth was still popular after the Han. A story in the *Sanguozhi*, quoting the *Lieyizhuan* 列異傳, told that when Hua Xin 華歆 was an examination candidate, he "once spent the night outside someone's house and the master's wife gave birth that night." Thus, delivery did not always mean being sent away. See *Sanguozhi*, 13.405. If one accepts the above-quoted explanation by Du Yu's commentary on "both emerged" as "emerged from the delivery house," then one might be able to use this as evidence for the practice in the Jin dynasty.

210 *Fengsu tongyi jiaozhu*, 562.

211 For information on valuing sons more than daughters in the Han, see Liu Zenggui (Tseng-kuei Liu) 劉增貴, *Handai hunyin zhidu* 漢代婚姻制度 (Taipei: Huashi chubanshe, 1982), 21; and Li Zhende, "Han Sui zhijian de 'shengzi buju' wenti," 759-60. The above-quoted story of the wife of Zhou Ba who exchanged her daughter for a butcher's son showed the pressure on women to give birth to sons, caused by the belief in ancestral worship in a patriarchal society. One can also cite the above-mentioned Empress Zhangsun of the Tang who sacrificed her life in order to ensure the continuation of the imperial line.

special birth room, either inside the house or outside. If it was inside, it would be like the *Liji* description: "[When] a wife is about to deliver a child, once [she has] entered the month, lodge her in a side room." Thus, after a woman entered the last month of pregnancy, a room was selected for her as the birth room, separate from the main sleeping rooms such as the actual bedroom or rooms for resting.[212] If the room was outside, it may have been constructed, as the *Chanjing* said, in a location relatively far from wells and stoves, with the goal of avoiding "great misfortune."

The inauspiciousness of childbirth stemmed primarily from the pollution inherent in the blood and fluids of delivery, which could easily lead to transgressions of taboos and offenses against the spirits. The Dunhuang text *Fumu enzhongjing jiangjingwen* 父母恩重經講經文 (Sermons on the sutra on the profound kindness of parents) describes the scene of women giving birth as "just like slaughtering pigs and goats, the blood flows so much that it covers the ground."[213] As quoted above, the *Chanjing* and the *Waitai miyao* both suggest methods such as spreading straw and sprinkling ashes, laying out the skin of a wild animal, or containing the blood and substances in a bowl to avoid breaking the taboo against blood and water touching the ground. The *Chanjing* also recommended reading out an invocation while spreading the straw, asking various spirits "to come here and protect me" and not allowing the "various evils to approach near."[214] The *Zimu milu* 子母祕錄 (Secret records of sons and mothers) of the Tang contained methods for "borrowing land" and "restraining the fluids," which helped the woman in labor "borrow a square of land from the various spirits" at the time of delivery.[215] At the same time, chanting an invocation while saving all the liquids used for cleaning and rinsing her meant to "use the clean to grasp the foul."[216] When the *Waitai miyao* quoted Cui Zhiti's birth chart, it also explained how to avoid the location of various spirits. The spirits' images indicated extreme powers, including the ability to protect the woman in labor and the force to injure if they were offended.

---

[212] *Liji*, 28.11a.

[213] Wang Zhongming 王重民, Wang Qingshu 王慶菽, Xiang Da 向達, Zhou Yiliang, Qi Gong 啓功, and Zeng Yigong 曾毅公, eds., *Dunhuang bianwenji* 敦煌變文集 (Beijing: Renmin wenxue chubanshe, 1984), B, vol. 5, 679, 699.

[214] *Ishinpo*, 23.8b

[215] *Ishinpo*, 23.7b-8a.

[216] *Ishinpo*, 23.8b-9a, quoting the *Zimu milu*.

The Daoist text *Yuanshitianzun jidu xuehu zhenjing* 元始天尊濟度血湖真經 (Authentic canon of salvation of the grand beginning Heavenly reverence; herafter cited as *Xuehu Zhenjing*) described the hell of Blood Lake, explaining that men and women who had offended the spirits would descend to this hell. According to its remarks, it was almost impossible for a married woman to avoid the worst fate:

> Childbirth entails various hardships. Maybe during their monthly flow they wash their dirty clothes. Maybe during childbirth their blood pollutes the ground. The polluted fluid is poured out into streams, rivers, ponds, and wells, and people of the world, without knowing it, draw water for drink and food and offer it as sacrifice to the spirits, thus offending the Three Illuminaries.... Maybe the child dies in the abdomen or the mother perishes after the birth, or both mother and child pass away, causing harm to lives.... With unexpected harm and unwanted destiny, she dies and enters the hell of Fengdu 酆都, suffering all sorts of torments. The lake is created from accumulated blood, and the hell exists because it recognizes the illusion of fate.... The *Yuanshitianzun* says, "I observe all the sentient creatures on earth. [When] women amass numerous sorts of sins, their bodies fall into Blood Lake and suffer, and they sink down for the duration of millions of millions of kalpas, never reaching the time to escape. I now open the enlightened box of the treasurehouse and issue the pardoning text of the golden scriptures....."[217]

The various measures recommended in the *Chanjing* were for the most part limited to specific taboo days or months such as "opposing the branch." The *Waitai miyao* also states explicitly that the purpose of all preparations was to prevent "the child dying in the abdomen or the delivery not going smoothly." The primary focus of the medical texts was to protect the mother and her fetus, and the targets and times of precautions were explicitly spelled out. The explanation in the *Xuehu zhenjing* for women's descent to the Blood Lake hell, however, not only expressed the strong aversion to substances expelled from female bodies but also revealed that, whether because of their reproductive duties or their household responsibilities, women were destined to take the blame, and there was no escape for them.

The discrepancies between the *Chanjing* and the *Xuehu zhenjing* might be due to the fact that prescription literature and Daoist literature were composed for different purposes, or that the later the

[217] *Yuanshitianzun jidu xuehu zhenjing, Zhengtong daozang dongzhenbu(su)* 正統道藏洞真部(宿) (Shanghai: Hanfenlou reprint of the Ming edition from Beijing Baiyun Daoist temple, 1924-26), vol. 32, juan A, 3-4, juan B.2.

date, the more clearly women's predicament was expressed.[218] The prescription literature did not explicitly blame women, but the numerous measures to prevent breaking taboos and offending the spirits conveyed a shared idea with the religious texts that women were impure due to their social roles while at the same time attempting to save them from childbirth complications.

Since the power of her impurity did not stop even after the conclusion of her delivery, the activities of a parturient woman received severe limitations accordingly. The taboo that prohibited women in childbirth from seeing other people existed from the Han dynasty on. The *Shenxianzhuan* 神仙傳 (Biography of immortals) described the scene when the female Immortal Magu 麻姑 paid a visit to Cai Jing's 蔡經 mother and the wife of Jing's younger brother: "The younger brother's wife had given birth more than ten days ago. When Magu looked up and saw her, she said, 'Ah, stop there, do not advance!'"[219] Having given birth more than ten days before still fell within the restrictions of the taboo. In the quotation above, Wang Chong described the custom in Jiangnan in which women in childbirth were so abhorred and avoided that they "are only allowed to enter after having passed through the month." The *Xiaopinfang* specifically stresses that what was called "fulfilling the month" in fact referred not merely to thirty days, the most important reason being that the mother's "body is experiencing an invisible pollution, and the lochia is not yet exhausted."

In addition to the filth and pollution of the blood of delivery and the lochia, women's childbirth-related impurity might have also been caused by the change of the her roles in the family. In traditional Chinese society, the most important function for women was

---

[218] Ren Jiyu 任繼愈, ed., *Daozang tiyao* 道藏提要 (Beijing: Zhongguo shehui kexue chubanshe, 1991), 55, states that this scripture "borrowed the name of the Yuanshitianzun to speak for the various transcendents." The name of the deity "Yuanshitianzun" was first seen in Tao Hongjing's *Zhenling weiyetu* 真靈位業圖 from the Southern Dynasties, and the practice of borrowing the name of the deity as author of Daoist scriptures gained popularity in the Tang dynasty. Scholars disagree on the date of the *Yuanshitianzun jidu xuehu zhenjing*, but some suggest the transition between Tang and Song. See Michel Soymié, "Tsubonkei no shiryoteki kenkyu," 血盆経の資料的研究, in Yoshioka Yoshitoyo and Michel Soymié, eds., *Dōkyō kennkyu* 道教研究 (Tokyo: Shoshinsha, 1965), 109-66. For a discussion of the Three Illuminaries in the Daoist Canon, see Chen Guofu 陳國符, *Daozang yuanliukao* 道藏源流考 (Beijing: Zhonghua shuju, 1963), 4-7.

[219] *Taiping yulan*, 803.6b.

to get married and bear sons in order to increase the number of descendants and continue the ancestral line of the husband's family. The lack of sons was a standard reason for men to expel a wife or to take a concubine, and on the basis of giving birth, a woman changed from being a wife and daughter-in-law to a mother, thus securing for herself a safe position in her husband's family. Childbirth was obviously the major turning point in this change in her status. Scholars have shown that human societies, when faced with this kind of shift in roles and relationships, frequently view it as a kind of "loss of order" or "impurity" and therefore enforce a period of isolation on the main actor.[220] The *Youyang zazu* 酉陽雜俎 (Miscellaneous morsels from Youyang) described "a wedding ritual from the Northern Dynasties: a space was made from a blue cloth screen, indoors or outdoors, which was called 'blue tent,' and in this [the couple] bowed to each other." Marriage was also an important ritual signifying a change of roles in life, and this wedding ritual also seemed to have the meaning of manifesting isolation in the temporary loss of order. Besides preventing exposure to wind, the practices of setting up a tent and erecting a screen found in early Chinese medical literature might have also expressed the message of the parturient woman's changing status in society. If this was so, then women's impurity was not only caused by the filth and foulness of the blood of childbirth, but was also related to the fact that childbirth carried the significance of re-forming family relationships.[221]

---

[220] See Van Gennep, *The Rites of Passage*, English trans. by Monika B. Vizedom and Gabrielle L. Caffee (Chicago: University of Chicago Press, 1960), 10-11, 191; Emily M. Ahern, "The Power and Pollution of Chinese Women," in Roxanne Witke and Margery Wolf, eds., *Women in Chinese Society* (Stanford: Stanford University Press, 1975), 199, 207.

[221] Anthropologists researching modern Chinese society also point out that women in patriarchal society may have formed intimate bonds and alliances with their sons that constituted possible threats to the patriarchal system. Therefore, giving birth, on the one hand, allowed women to make a contribution to the continuation of the ancestral line, but, on the other hand, it gave them the destructive power to disrupt the order of the patriarchal system. The taboos and regulations against this sort of "loss of order" also were a factor in regarding women in childbirth as "impure" or "inauspicious" as well as enforcing their isolation. For a discussion, see Ahern, "The Power and Pollution of Chinese Women," 199, 207. Research on the social aspects of ancient Chinese concepts of impurity has been scarce up to now. Please see discussion by Edward Schafer, "The Development of Bathing Customs in Ancient and Medieval China and the History of the Floriate Clear Palace," *Journal of American Oriental Society* 76.2 (1956): 57-82, and Robin Yates, "Purity and Pollution in Early China," in Tsang

Conclusion

From ancient times on, childbirth was a matter of life or death. For the woman giving birth, it was a question of survival or perishing, and for her family, an opportunity for failure or success. In early imperial China, doctors warned against women marrying and bearing children too early, but customs were hard to change. Faced with the serious event of childbirth, people responded in certain ways when entering the month, during delivery, and postpartum. The specific month for ingesting medicinal decoctions to make the fetus slippery was not clearly defined before the seventh century, but after the Tang-Song period, the time for ingesting each type of medicinal decoction had been gradually determined. From the perspective of the inauspiciousness of childbirth, it was not easy to choose a place for delivery. Sending the woman away for the delivery and erecting a tent were actions performed with the purpose of isolation, in order to find an appropriate place for the woman to deliver. Before the Tang, the delivery might have occured indoors or outdoors, but in most cases a tent was set up in order to avoid Wind evil. The birth was performed according to birth charts, which prescribed setting up a screen, erecting a tent, the squatting position, and the burial of the placenta. By the seventh century, birth charts seemed to have undergone a process of integration, having been reduced and systematized from separate categories into one chart. Differences between rich and poor were most apparent in prenatal preparations and postpartum care. But when the time of delivery arrived, people probably combined a variety of different treatments, regardless of their social status, all with the goal of smooth delivery and speedy results.

Cheng-hwa 臧振華 ed., *Zhongguo kaoguxue yu lishixue zhi zhenghe yanjiu* 中國考古學與歷史學之整合研究 (Taipei: Institute of History and Philosophy, Academia Sinica, 1997), 479-536. As for recent research on the mother-and-son relationship in early imperial China, see Simomi Takao下見隆雄, *Jukyō shakai to bosei: bosei no iryoku no kanten de miru Kan Gi Shin Chugoku jyoseisi* 儒教社会と母性：母性の威力の観点でみる漢魏晋中国女性史 (Tokyo: Kenbun syuban, 1994); Alan Cole, *Mothers and Sons in Chinese Buddhism* (Stanford: Stanford University Press, 1998); and Zheng Yaru (Ya-ju Cheng) 鄭雅如, "Qinggan yu zhidu: Wei Jin shiqi de muziguansi" 情感與制度：魏晉時期的母子關係, in the *Wenshi congkan* series 文史叢刊 (Taipei: College of Liberal Arts, National Taiwan University, 2001).

During delivery, women clung to ropes, leaned in a vertical position, or were supported by others around the waist. Because of the ideal that "a smooth birth was fast and with little pain," the birth assistants might have alarmed the woman in labor with their activities or restrained her in disorderly ways. In their explanations for childbirth complications, doctors in early imperial China went beyond transgressed taboos and offended spirits. Moreover, they were already aware of the treatment of transverse and breech presentation by poking the fetus to make it recoil in order to turn around to the right position. And the procedures for treating childbirth complications show that people believed in such ideas as responding as early as possible for prevention, using various treatments in combination, and the mutual correspondence of substances. The husband was seen as a responsible party and not a bystander, while the participation of the community might have differed depending on time and place. During the final stage of labor, relatives and friends were likely to gather as birth assistants and express their opinions, which may have also influenced the process of birth for the parturient woman. Male doctors not only blamed birth assistants for their inappropriate actions, but sometimes even suggested that they were altogether unnecessary. Because female birth assistants have not had their own voice in the past and male doctors were summoned mostly in the case of complications only, the mutual appreciation or animosity between these two parties was bound to become a point of argument in both medical and women's history.

When the fetus and the placenta had been completely expelled, this meant that an important stage of the parturient woman's suffering was completed, but she was forced to remain isolated from her regular daily life for a while longer, owing to ideas about avoiding Wind evil and the inauspiciousness of childbirth. The woman was considered impure due to such factors as the pollution of blood and lochia as well as her changed social role. In elite families, women in childbed might have been able to enjoy more than a month of rest, because of ideas in the medical texts regarding the need to heal injuries and replenish deficiencies. The mistress of a nuclear peasant family, however, probably had to get back to work not long after the birth. At any rate, friends and relatives would come to congratulate, bringing nurturing and replenishing foods. Doctors referred to the gifts as "tonifying and nurturing the five internal [organs], not for celebrating her child." They encouraged women to marry late and bear fewer children in order to prevent "blood withering which could cause death." This should probably indicate the concern for the female body as such, in addition to her function as a reproductive vessel.

Review Article

DEPLETED MEN, EMOTIONAL WOMEN: GENDER AND MEDICINE IN THE MING DYNASTY

BY

MARTA E. HANSON
(Johns Hopkins University)

Joanna Grant. *A Chinese Physician: Wang Ji and the 'Stone Mountain Medical Case Histories.'* Needham Research Institute Series. London: Routledge Curzon, 2003. xi, 209 pp., illus. £55.00/US$114.95 cloth. ISBN 0-415-29758-3.

General Assessments

In her new book *Vernacular Bodies*, Mary Fissell asks questions broadly relevant for the history of women, gender, and medicine anywhere. How did ordinary people understand the female body in early modern England, and what are the broader implications of changes in their understanding? She used vernacular sources—ballads, jokes, images, pamphlets, broadsides, and popular medical manuals—instead of elite medical treatises to demonstrate how women's bodies had became a cultural site for the articulation and discussion of historical changes, specifically the Protestant Reformation and the English Civil War.[1] Changes in the meanings of women's bodies did not just reflect historic moments, but rather these interpretations of female bodies were the way ordinary people made meaning of and worked out the crises in gender relations integral to both periods.[2] The "world turned upside down" during the English Civil War, for instance,

[1] Mary E. Fissell, *Vernacular Bodies: The Politics of Reproduction in Early Modern England* (Oxford: Oxford University Press, 2004).

[2] For other methodological insights useful for the history of gender, women, and medicine in China, see Mary E. Fissell, "Making Meaning from the Margins: The New Cultural History of Medicine," in Frank Huisman and John Harley Warner, eds., *Locating Medical History: The Stories and Their Meanings* (Baltimore: Johns Hopkins University Press, 2004), 364-89.

precipitated a broad crisis in paternity and a concomitant assertion of male authority over female bodies and of male involvement in reproduction.

Using elite instead of vernacular sources in Chinese medical history, both Francesca Bray and Charlotte Furth have similarly shown how medical authors worked out crises in gender relations, social changes, and economic transformations through reinterpretations of reproduction and the female body.[3] Yet, discourses on female bodies in both England and China were as much about men as they were about women and perhaps even more about political crises and social ills than illness per se. The most recent and interesting study of this phenomenon in China is Joanna Grant's gender analysis of the case records of an elite Chinese physician named Wang Ji 汪機 (1463-1539). Grant finds the locus of gender anxiety in male instead of female bodies. She reads Wang's dominant diagnoses of male corporeal depletion as an extension of his moral concern about the excesses of pleasure and consumption of his era. Wary of the immoral behaviors and high social aspirations of the newly emergent merchant class in his native Huizhou 徽州 region, Wang responded to the social ills of his day by treating what he perceived to be the resulting depletion disorders in his male patients. He advocated warming and replenishing drugs to boost the protective system he thought his upwardly mobile male clients had worn down through excessive sex, food, and wine. Here we see how male more than female bodies became a cultural site for Wang Ji's articulation of and response to the dramatic economic, social, and cultural changes in the Huizhou region during his lifetime.

Grant's case study is intended not just for historians of Chinese medicine and historians of medicine elsewhere, but also for historians of late imperial China, especially those interested in gender and women in Chinese history. By focusing on a specific time, place, and physician, she astutely connects the economic, social, and cultural

[3] Charlotte Furth, *A Flourishing Yin: Gender in China's Medical History, 960-1665* (Berkeley: University of California Press, 1999). Francesca Bray, *Technology and Gender: Fabrics of Power in Late Imperial China* (Berkeley: University of California Press, 1997). Fissell cites both in *Vernacular Bodies*, 13. Literate Chinese medical conceptions of reproduction were considerably sophisticated. See also Angela Ki Che Leung, "Autour de la naissance: La mère et l'enfant en Chine aux XVIe et XVIIe siècles," *Cahiers internationaux de sociologie* 76 (1984):51-69.

transformations in late fifteenth and early sixteenth-century Huizhou with the medical concerns of Wang Ji, arguably the most successful and prolific *ruyi* 儒醫 (literati physician) of his time.[4]

The structure of *A Chinese Physician* follows three explicit methodologies: traditional socioeconomic and biographic, textual, and gender analyses. The traditional socioeconomic and biographic method guides the opening chapter in which Wang Ji emerges as an upright Confucian gentleman who, having failed in the civil service examinations, turned to medicine as an alternative means to benefit society, and, presumably to make a living. His disciples collected over one hundred of his cases, compiled them into one text, and published them in 1531 as the *Shishan yi'an* 石山醫案 (Stone Mountain medical case histories).[5] Their compilation is the earliest extant Chinese medical text devoted to the clinical encounters of one physician.[6]

The textual analysis begins in the second chapter, which covers the history of the *yi'an* as a genre and the contents of the *Stone Mountain* text itself. *Stone Mountain* contains not only Wang's case histories but also those of physicians who supported his views, several doctrinal essays, and two biographies, one of him and the other one by him of his father, who was also a physician. Grant argues that Wang did not mention marginal, folk, or female healers, engaging exclusively with issues that concerned other elite male physicians. This new medical genre of case histories used the model of legal cases to secure a place for Wang's views in the contemporary medical debates made available through the sixteenth-century boom in medical

[4] See my first review of *A Chinese Physician,* by Marta Hanson, *Medical History* 48.1 (2004):397-99. Ordinarily, I would not review a book twice, but in this case, I have delved deeper into the Chinese evidence and changed my original assessment of the conclusions.

[5] For a modern edition of this book, I use the collection of Wang Ji's medical texts in the *Ming Qing mingyi quanshu dacheng* 明清名醫全書大成 (Compilation of the complete works of famous physicians from the Ming and Qing) series. Gao Erxin 高爾鑫, ed., *Wang Shishan Yixue quanshu* 汪石山醫學全書 (Beijing: Zhongguo zhongyiyao chubanshe, 1999).

[6] See Nathan Sivin on the political context and clinical contents of the earliest medical histories from the Han dynasty in "Text and Experience in Classical Chinese Medicine," in Don Bates, ed., *Knowledge and the Scholarly Medical Traditions* (Cambridge: Cambridge University Press, 1995), 177-204; and Christopher Cullen on the history of the genre thereafter, "*Yi'an* (case statements): Origins of a Genre of Chinese Medical Literature," in Elisabeth Hsu, ed., *Innovation in Chinese Medicine* (Cambridge: Cambridge University Press, 2001), 297-323.

publishing.[7] Wang and his disciples chose cases that demonstrated the efficacy of his preference for replenishing tonics to treat cases of *qi* 氣 depletion. The third chapter continues the textual analysis by exploring Wang's theoretical positions and therapeutic preferences through his clinical encounters, the doctor-patient dynamic, and evidence of competitors.

Although gender is mentioned throughout the first three chapters, the core of the gender analysis is in the final chapter on gender, culture, and medicine. Here Grant examines when gender did and did not matter in the 109 cases traced directly to Wang Ji of more than 170 case histories discussed in *Stone Mountain*.[8] By looking at both sexes as well as the full range of female disorders within one collection of medical histories, Grant expands upon the scholarship of her predecessors and challenges previous conclusions.[9]

One reviewer has already assessed the ways in which Grant's socioeconomic analysis could be improved. Not only did disruptive changes in Huizhou culture and commerce influence Wang Ji's dominant medical diagnosis of male depletion, but also the comparatively strong devotion to Confucian education in the Huizhou region and internalization of Confucian classics such as the *Yijing* 易經 (Book of Changes) may have influenced Wang's medical theory as much as did his professional identity as a *ruyi* literati physician. Similarly, within the Huizhou context of merchant families investing in their sons' education for success in the civil service examinations, the tension evoked between upright Confucian physicians and wayward

[7] On the growth of medical publishing during the late Ming to early Qing transition, see Ellen Widmer, "The *Huanduzhai* of Hangzhou and Suzhou: A Study in Seventeenth-century Publishing," *Harvard Journal of Asiatic Studies* 56.1 (1996):77-122. For medical publishing in the Huizhou region, see Marta Hanson, "Merchants of Medicine: Huizhou Mercantile Consciousness, Morality, and Medical Patronage in Seventeenth-century China," in Keizo Hashimoto, Catherine Jami, and Lowell Skar, eds., *East Asian Science: Tradition and Beyond* (Osaka: Kansai University Press, 1995), 207-14.

[8] The additional sixty-one case histories were of children or attributed to other physicians. For evidence from the primary sources, see Gao Erxin ed., *Wang Shishan Yixue quanshu* (1999).

[9] She particularly engages with Charlotte Furth's first two articles: "Blood, Body, and Gender: Medical Images of the Female Condition in China," *Chinese Science* 7 (1986):43-66; and "Concepts of Pregnancy, Childbirth, and Infancy in Ch'ing Dynasty China," *Journal of Asian Studies* 46.1 (1987):7-35.

Huizhou merchants may have been more imagined among literati than real in society.[10]

Another reviewer raises several issues with Grant's argument that Wang had unique medical perspectives and that they are best explained as the product of culture.[11] If the literati backlash against the perceived decadence of the Huizhou *nouveau riche* was widespread, one should be able to find comparable cultural effects on the medical practices of other Huizhou physicians. Wang also may not have been as much of an iconoclast as an innovator within a newly emerging doctrinal lineage from Li Gao 李杲 (1180-1251) and Zhu Zhenheng 朱震亨 (1281-1358) to his contemporary Xue Ji 薛己 (1487-1559), the leading proponent of the *wenbu* 溫補 (warm replenishing) therapeutic doctrine, which Wang Ji strongly favored. Moreover, Furth had previously shown that other sixteenth-century authors of *fuke* 婦科 (gynecology) texts appear to be similarly more interested in male self-cultivation practices to ensure fertility and fecundity than in the female differences that preoccupied earlier *fuke* authors since the Song.[12] Because Grant's socioeconomic and cultural interpretations have already been sufficiently assessed, this review focuses instead on the gender analysis of the medical case histories presented in the final chapter.

Three methodological weaknesses mitigate the persuasiveness of Grant's claims. These cracks in the edifice relate to the presentation and interpretation of primary evidence, the limitation of relying on only one text of a prolific physician's corpus without broadly reading his views on male and female differences, and a limited use of gender analysis that tends to challenge more than further previous scholarship. This critique generally follows the structure of the gender analysis chapter, with general facts and figures followed by sections on diagnosis, etiology, illness syndrome, treatment, and outcome.

---

[10] See the review of *A Chinese Physician* by Ann Shu-ju Chiu, *East Asian Science Technology and Medicine* 21 (2003):156-61. For evidence of the renewed relations between the literati and merchants in the Ming-Qing period using mostly sources on Huizhou, see Yu Yingshi 余英時, *Zhongguo jinshi zongjiao lunli yu shangren jingshen* 中國近世宗教倫理與商人精神 (Taibei: Lianjing Publishers, 1987).

[11] For the criticisms and insights on Grant's cultural interpretation summarized here, see the review of *A Chinese Physician* by Yi-Li Wu, *Journal of Asian Studies* 64.2 (2005):442-4.

[12] See Furth, *A Flourishing Yin*, Ch. 6, "Nourishing Life," 187-206.

Facts and Figures

First, let us do the numbers. Although most of the claims rely on them, they are incomplete and unnecessarily confusing. Grant focuses her analysis on 109 of the 123 cases attributed to Wang Ji in the three fascicles of *Stone Mountain*, the other 14 being either of children or from other physicians. Table 4.1 on disorder classifications, however, includes the cases histories of children and from other physicians. It also lists the number of men (67, including 5 children and 3 supplementary cases) and women (38, including 1 child and 2 supplementary cases) for the thirty classifications of disorders in the first two fascicles. The unnecessary confusion stems from Grant's choice not to include in Table 4.1 either the twenty-two other classes of disorders or the fourteen cases (10 male, 4 female listed in Table 4.2) from the third fascicle.[13] Table 4.2 then presents the distribution of the 109 cases (68 male, 41 female) attributed to Wang Ji in all three fascicles, excluding the case histories of children or from other physicians. Not only do the totals of male and female cases in Tables 4.1 and 4.2 not match, but also because data from the third fascicle was left out of Table 4.1, the gender distribution of the twenty-two diagnoses for the remaining fourteen cases (actually twenty-one) in the third fascicle cannot be known without checking the Chinese original. The reader or reviewer should not have to do this additional work. Grant explains her choice by stating that "cases in the third fascicle are not arranged according to any definable pattern" (p. 105), but does not give further details about its contents. It is always better to err on the side of caution and present all available data in a consistent way. By choosing to excise data because it did not fit an obvious pattern, Grant not only risked criticisms of data manipulation, but also lost the opportunity to see the underlying logic of the original author.

Table 4.2 divides Wang's 109 cases according to male and female in each of the three fascicles. This division reveals a much higher proportion of female cases in the second fascicle (24 male/22 female, 52%/48%), then in the first (34 male/15 female, 70%/30%)

---

[13] Although in Table 4.2, Grant lists ten male and four female patients for the third fascicle, the fascicle refers to twenty-one cases, fifteen male and six female. Grant excluded five of the fifteen male cases and two of the six female cases because Wang did not see them himself.

and third fascicles (10 male/4 female 71%/29%). This discrepancy is due to the four sections in the second fascicle that group together female disorders related to menstruation, irregular pulses, pregnancy, and postnatal problems. Although the overall sex ratio of the 109 cases was 1.7 male to 1 female, when the reproductive cases were excluded, Table 4.2 demonstrates that the other two fascicles contained similar sex ratios of approximately 2.3 males to 1 female case. Wang Ji clearly saw more male than female patients, but he also had a significant percentage of female patients who saw him for nonreproductive problems. Grant concurs with other scholars that Chinese women were most likely first to see female rather than male healers[14] and only sought male physicians as a last resort. She casts light for the first time, however, on an important distinction between reproductive and nonreproductive disorders among the female cases.

As a result, Table 4.3 divides the forty-one cases of Wang's mature female patients from all three fascicles into three categories based on the type of relation between the main disorder and reproduction: A) seventeen women or 41 percent had disorders unrelated to reproduction, B) nine women or 22 percent had disorders not directly related to reproduction but complicated by a recent pregnancy or birth, and C) fifteen women or 37 percent suffered explicitly from reproductive disorders related to menstruation, pregnancy, pulse abnormalities, and postnatal conditions. About two thirds of Wang's female patients suffered from nonreproductive disorders.

Grant argues convincingly that one should look at the full range of illnesses among Chinese women to better understand how gender played out in the clinical encounter, diagnosis, and treatment. She makes two arguments related to this position. In contrast to the emphasis on reproductive disorders and menstrual regularity found in

[14] Grant contradicts herself on female healers. First she discusses "the only example in the *Shishan yi'an* of a female healer of any sort" (98-99) and then she writes that "There is evidence from contemporaneous sources, both historical and literary, to substantiate this explanation, although there is no mention of female healers in the *Shishan yi'an* itself" (107). The essay on *si* 思 (pensiveness) in the third fascicle, however, mentions a *nuwu* 女巫 (female spirit medium) hired by a husband to help him cure his wife of unceasing grief after her mother's death. See *Wang Shishan Yixue quanshu: Shishan yi'an* (*juan* 3), 98b. Nathan Sivin translates the same case in the article "Emotional Counter-Therapy," *Medicine, Philosophy and Religion in Ancient China* (England: Variorum, 1995), 11.

Chinese gynecological texts, Wang Ji did not consider menses integral to his diagnosis of female patients suffering from nonreproductive problems. He did not, in other words, always follow the maxim "ruled by Blood" that Furth found to be dominantly the case in *fuke* texts after the Song dynasty.[15] Nor did he consider his female patients to be ruled by their uterus, as many of his Western medical contemporaries would have assumed.[16]

Grant did not consider, however, the ages of these women. Wang, on the other hand, considered age important enough to state it directly after the sex of most of his male and female patients. Of the seventeen women with nonreproductive disorders, for example, seven are over fifty years old, three are over forty, three are over thirty, one just turned thirty, and three have no age stated.[17] Ten of the women with nonreproductive disorders (58 percent) were over forty years old when Wang saw them. Wang Ji may not have mentioned their menses or indicated any reproductive complications simply because they were obviously past their reproductive years. This could have also been the case for the women in their thirties since Ming women tended to marry young and begin reproducing in their late teens and early twenties.

Furthermore, Wang gave the ages of his female patients more frequently for class A cases of nonreproductive disorders (fourteen out of seventeen) than either class B cases of nonreproductive disorders complicated by pregnancy or birth (two out of nine, of which both women were over thirty) or class C cases, when the women clearly had reproductive disorders (five out of fifteen, of which two were in their twenties, two were over forty, and one was fifty-two years old). All fourteen of the ages given for the seventeen nonreproductive cases in class A, in fact, were for middle-aged women between thirty and fifty years old. This evidence suggests that age was central in Wang's clinical assessment of his female patients and was di-

---

[15] I refer here to Furth, *A Flourishing Yin*.

[16] For an overview of the relation between the uterus and hysteria in Western medical history, see Ilza Veith, *Hysteria: The History of a Disease* (Chicago: University of Chicago Press, 1965).

[17] The three women for whom an age was not given suffered from ailments unrelated to reproduction: *shenma* 身麻 (numbness) from sitting too long and *jiaochuang* 脚瘡 (foot sores), nevertheless related to irregular menses, and *si* (pensiveness) over the death of her mother (see n. 13). For the cases, see *Shishan yi'an* in *Wang Shishan Yixue quanshu*, 78b, 87a, 98b.

rectly related to his sense of their reproductive status. One sees this clearly in his medical views on virgins and widows.

Reading Beyond the "Stone Mountain Case Histories"

Women in class A who had reached menopause would have been considered no longer predisposed toward *yin* or Blood depletion but rather susceptible to the opposite. In one compilation titled *Waike li li* 外科理例 (Patterns and examples for external medicine; preface, 1531), Wang wrote an unusual essay about widows titled *Lun guafu bing jiushiwu* 論寡婦病九十五 (On widows' disorders no. 95). For Wang, menopause occurred among widows because they no longer had an outlet for their sexual desire and suffered exhaustion from exuberant Blood (*xuesheng* 血盛), the opposite of Blood depletion:

> They live alone without *yang*; they desire a man, but because they cannot obtain one, they get depressed and become ill. They dwell in the women's quarters where they have desire but no way to fulfill it. *Yin* and *yang* struggle, hot and cold alternate, just like the class of intermittent fevers. After a while, this causes them to become exhausted and acquire syndromes such as amenorrhea, white flux, phlegm, dizziness, *qi* in the diaphragm, abdominal lumps, facial discoloration, and emaciation, all of which are illnesses of widows. Feeling their pulse, they only have a stringy Liver pulse, which comes out of the "Inch Opening" (*cunkou* 寸口) [on the inside of the wrist] and rises to the "Fish border" (*yuji* 魚際) [point on the inside base joint of the thumb], all of which indicate exuberant Blood.[18] The *Inner Canon* says: Men who have exuberant Essence [*qi*] think of taking a wife; women who have exuberant Blood conceive.[19]

We see here that Blood was as central to Wang's understanding of the special pathologies of widows as it was in his essays on menses and reproductive disorders. His essay *Yuejing men* 月經門 (Menstruation), for example, predictably begins with the statement: "Women are *yin* and take Blood as their root."[20]

Wang discusses widows in another essay from the same book titled *Lun jing xue bashiqi* 論精血八十七 (On essence and Blood no. 87).

---

[18] The "Inch Opening" is the location of the wrist pulse closest to the base of the wrist. The "Fish Border" is the LU-10 point located on the Lung channel. It is located in a depression behind the base joint of the thumb between the midpoint of the shaft of the first metacarpal bone and the thenar muscles.

[19] *Waike li li*: *Lun guifu bing jiushiwu* (*juan* 2) in *Wang Shishan Yixue quanshu*, 380a-b.

[20] *Yixue yuanli*: *Yuejing men* (*juan* 12) in *Wang Shishan Yixue quanshu*, 813a-b.

This time he links both the lack of sexual intercourse and the lack of sexual desire with amenorrhea: "As for women whose menses have ceased, they stop when they have either not had intercourse with a man for ten years or have not thought about sex with a man for ten years. If the menses do not flow, then the old Blood cannot exit, the new Blood flows in the wrong direction, sometimes leaking into the bones and sometimes transforming and causing swelling. If they do have sex, it is difficult for them to have children."[21]

One of his widowed patients over forty fit these criteria. Wang discussed her *xuebeng* 血崩 (profuse uterine bleeding) in the longest case under *Tiaojing* 調經 (Regulating menstruation) in *Stone Mountain*.[22] Wang clearly indicates that she has been widowed for over ten years, which according to "On widows' disorders" puts her at risk for exuberant Blood. Instead of the bitter and cold drugs intended to stop the excessive abnormal bleeding that other physicians prescribed, however, Wang prescribed his preferred warming and replenishing herbs to treat an underlying spleen and stomach *qi* depletion. After being cured, however, the widow took a long trip to her natal home by sedan chair. Completely exhausted from this trip, she experienced an even more severe case of uterine bleeding. Wang wrote that "After fifty years, the Blood and *qi* slip out [of their normal channels], so actually it was hard to save [her] life, but I could not bear to sit and watch her die."[23] He gave her a strong dose of mostly ginseng and astragalus root, with some of his other preferred herbs, and she recovered.[24] Here again we see that Wang Ji considered age an important factor in the balance of Blood and *qi* in relation to the life stages of his female patients.

In the previous essay "On widows' disorders no. 95," Wang also compares the effect of repressed sexual desire on depleted Essence in virgin boys and depleted Blood in virgin girls: "For a boy, first

[21] *Waike li li*: *Lun jing xue bashiqi* (*juan* 2) in *Wang Shishan*, *Yixue quanshu*, 379a-b.

[22] *Shishan yi'an*: *Tiaojing* (*juan* 2) in *Wang Shishan Yixue quanshu*, 88b-90a.

[23] *Shishan yi'an*: *Tiaojing* (*juan* 2) in *Wang Shishan Yixue quanshu*, 89b.

[24] He prescribed seven *qian* 錢 of ginseng and astragalus root, one *qian* of Chinese angelica root, rehmannia glutinosa, ginger, and cyperus tuber, and five *fen* 分 of licorice. Grant's section on treatment mentions four of these herbs—ginseng, astragalus, angelica, and licorice—as among the top five that formed the core of Wang's prescriptions, the fifth being atractylodes rhizome (p. 147).

his facial expression scatters; for a girl, first her period ceases."[25] Wang criticizes other physicians who do not know the appropriate prescriptions to start a virgin's period. They administer cold formulas because they wrongly assume that a virgin's Blood is classified as hot. Instead, doctors should know that Blood moves with heat and congeals with coolness. The symptoms of comparatively scant menses and no flow are aches in the hands, feet, bones, and flesh; waves of heat; a gradual wasting away; and a weak pulse. For Wang, all of these conditions indicate cases of Yin depletion and Blood deficiency, diagnoses dominantly gendered female in *fuke* texts. Because Blood requires heat to move, he recommends warm medicines to start the menses of virgins who have conditions of depleted Blood.[26] Whether at the beginning or the end of the reproductive life cycle of women, Blood still ruled women in Wang's theoretical essays as well as in cases of female disorders involving reproduction.

In several other essays in *Waike li li*, Wang also discusses how the sexes differ in terms of illnesses, emotions, and appropriate treatments. In an essay titled *Lun jiaoqi jiushiba* 論腳氣九十八 (On foot *qi* no. 98), Wang follows the Song physician Chen Ziming 陳自明 (1190-1270) on how *jiaoqi* 腳氣 (foot *qi*) differs between the sexes.[27] In the *fuke* section of the tenth-century Song pharmacopoeia *Taiping sheng hui fang* 太平聖惠方 (Imperial Grace formulary), for example, foot *qi* was classified as a disorder of the circulation channels associated with the womb. Chen Ziming linked it to weakness of the Kidney system for men and weakness in the channels of the womb for women.[28] Following this line of reasoning, Wang argues that although women as well as men suffer from it, they contract this illness because their "Sea of Blood has become deficient and they are affected by the seven emotions" and not from the gluttony or sexual wantonness to which men were more socially prone.[29] For men, foot *qi* is due to Kidney deficiency from sexual excess; for women, it is the result of Blood deficiency or emotional excess. The same medicine is used for men and women, but Wang warns that to treat

[25] See both essays *Lun jing xue bashiqi* and *Lun furen bing bashijiu*, in *Waike li li*, (*juan* 2) in *Wang Shishan Yixue quanshu*, 379.

[26] *Waike li li*: *Lun guifu bing jiushiwu* (*juan* 2) in *Wang Shishan Yixue quanshu*, 380.

[27] *Waike li li: Lun jiaoqi jiushijba* (*juan* 2) in *Wang Shishan Yixue quanshu*, 381.

[28] Furth discusses the gendered aspects of "foot *qi*" in *A Flourishing Yin*, 82-83, 166, 167 n. 18.

[29] *Waike li li*: *Lun jiaoqi jiushijba* (*juan* 2) in *Wang Shishan Yixue quanshu*, 381.

women effectively, the medicinal treatment must be combined with manipulation of the seven emotions.

Wang also quotes Zhu Zhenheng on sexual differences in temperaments in an essay titled *Nan nu yong ju zhifa butong ershiwu* 男女癰疽治法不同二十五 (On how the treatment method for swollen sores of the *yong* and *ju* type differs for men and women no. 25): "It is ten times more difficult to control the temperament of a woman than that of a man." This gender bias also appears in an essay *Lun funu bing bashijiu* 論婦女病八十九 (On women's disorders no. 89), which focuses on female susceptibility to emotions: "Women's temperament is to hold on to the emotions; they are not able to release them and are more often damaged by the seven emotions .... It is best first to give them Four-Seven decoction to regulate the draining *qi* and then use drugs that nourish the Blood."[30] In Wang's other medical writing, even more evidence of gender differences and the role of Blood in female pathology contradicts Grant's interpretations of the data.

A broader reading of his corpus on widows and virgins, for example, challenges Grant's claims that Wang did not consider Blood central in his distinctions of women at different stages of the reproductive cycle. Grant's dual emphases on the exceptions to the rule and fissures between theory and practice are methodologically useful and insightful. Exceptions to the rule that in Chinese medicine "Blood is the root for women" do not, however, necessarily override the general rule. Rather these exceptions illuminate how medical case histories reveal a greater complexity and flexibility within the clinical encounter than is otherwise preserved in doctrinal essays. With these insights from Grant's analysis in mind, we now turn to the clinical encounter.

Diagnosis

When Wang interviewed his patients, he followed the *sizhen* 四診 (four examinations) method of diagnosis: looking, listening/smelling, asking, and touching. Although he indicates the sex of the patient first, sex thereafter become largely irrelevant. One has a sense of

---

30 *Waike li li: Nan nü yongju zhifa butong ershisi* (*juan* 1) in *Wang Shishan Yixue quanshu*, 361.

greater similarity than difference. Grant argues that Wang did not routinely question women about menstruation and found no evidence that the information provided on women's menses was integral to diagnosis. Since menstruation did not appear to Grant to play a central role in Wang's female cases, she calls into question the centrality of menstrual regulation to female health in Chinese medicine. As already discussed, the age of the female patients may have been as much a factor in this omission as the nonreproductive nature of their complaints. This evidence nevertheless suggests that the medical view of women was not confined solely to their role as potential child bearers. Nevertheless, Wang more often than not indicated the reproductive status of his female patients somewhere in their medical case histories, whether through statements of their age or about their menses, and often both.

With respect to asking, Grant surprisingly found that Wang did not have any difficulty talking with his female patients. All seemed candid about their reproductive and nonreproductive problems, which contrasts markedly with work by other scholars.[31] Two women of means even came by sedan chair to visit him, which differs from accounts of other Ming physicians frustrated not only by women's inaccessibility, but also by the conventions of modesty required during house calls. The only difference Grant found was that Wang never quoted a woman replying to him or asking him about a diagnosis. He attributed speech only to men. With respect to touching, Wang took the pulses of both his female and male patients. The issue of gender and modesty so explicit in theoretical texts, and even in fiction, appears not to have been an issue in Wang's practice.[32] This contrast, Grant points out, may be because Wang was not as concerned with reproductive disorders as were many of his predecessors and contemporaries.[33] Another possibility relates back to the bias in the selection criteria toward successful treatments of *qi* de-

---

[31] I refer to the work of Cullen (1993), Bray (1997), and Furth (1986, 1987, 1999).

[32] For Ming examples, see Christopher Cullen, "Patients and Healers in Late Imperial China: Evidence from the *Jinpingmei*," *History of Science* 31 (1993):99-150. For comparable Qing evidence, see Yi-Li Wu, "The Bamboo Grove Monastery and Popular Gynecology in Qing China," *Late Imperial China* 21.1 (2000):41-76.

[33] See the chapter on the Yangzhou doctor Cheng Maoxian 程茂先 (1581-?) in Furth, *A Flourishing Yin*, 224-65.

pletion on which Wang staked his reputation and secured a legacy among his male and female patients.

Illness Syndromes and Treatments

Based on Wang's discussions of illnesses, Grant argues that there is no evidence that he found male and female bodies dissimilar in form, function, or processes. Nor did he address in the theoretical sections or case histories the differences in the nature of male and female bodies or in the way the two sexes react to illness. If Grant had read broadly in his medical writings, she would have found that Wang discussed these sexual differences elsewhere. Perhaps this was the case because such differences were irrelevant to the key arguments of *Stone Mountain*. The opening passage of the essay on *Yuejing men* (Menstruation) of his *Yixue yuanli* 醫學原理 (The first principles of medical learning) states: "Women are classified as *yin* and take Blood as the root. Humans resemble Heaven and Earth, and *yin* is often insufficient. Moreover, because of the diminishing [of *qi*] due to breast-feeding and menses in women, their *yin* and Blood are more deficient, which is the reason why most women suffer from Blood disorders."[34] Other passages on sexual differences cited above further illustrate the contradiction between what Grant found in the case histories and what Wang wrote about in his doctrinal essays.

To what extent did gender have an effect on Wang's choice of treatment? Grant argues again that the evidence shows that the main difference in therapy was not between men and women but between women with and without reproductive illnesses. He gave ginseng (*renshen* 人參) to nearly all his patients, male (80 percent) and female (70 percent), and another four replenishing drugs—atractylodes rhizome (*baishu* 白朮), Chinese angelica root (*danggui* 當歸), licorice (*gancao* 甘草), and astragalus root (*huangqi* 黃芪)—to two-thirds of the male and just one-half of the female patients. Men had a higher rate than women of depletion treated by these herbs. Although Wang prescribed cyperus tuber (*xiangfu* 香附) and donkey-hide gelatin (*ajiao* 阿膠) to more women than men because of their proper-

[34] Essay on menses, *Yixue yuanli*: *Yuejing men* (*juan* 12), in *Wang Shishan Yixue quanshu*, 813.

ties to regulate menstruation, replenish Blood, and stop bleeding, he did not use these drugs as much when his female patients had disorders unrelated to reproduction (p. 147).

Clinical Outcomes

In the final stage of the clinical encounter, Grant makes one of her boldest arguments. According to three criteria—overall recovery rates (90 percent male, 85 percent female), number of treatments required for recovery, and number of healers seen before Dr. Wang—she argues that contrary to the theoretical essays, in the case histories, women were neither sicker nor harder to treat than men. With just one treatment, for example, Wang cured 70 percent of female and 50 percent of male patients. After the second treatment, he cured another 20 percent of female and 30 percent of male patients. He cured as many men as women only after four treatments. With respect to number of healers, nearly three-fourths of the men and just three-fifths of the women saw more than one doctor. Not only did most women survive among Wang's patients, but they also recovered more quickly and saw fewer healers than men. By contrast, more men than women suffered from serious *yin* depletion, and men rather than women appear to have been the more difficult sex to treat.

What are we to make of these unexpected findings? Instead of the cultural analysis Grant employed to interpret Wang's cases of male depletion as cultural constructions based on perception of moral decay, Grant welds a social analysis grounded in demographic facts to the unexpected image of women as being healthier than men. Men may have had more access to physicians because of their greater mobility. A woman could only see an elite physician like Dr. Wang by going through her husband or son, making it less convenient for women than men to return. Women may have also chosen not to disclose visits with marginal and female healers, which based on evidence from mostly literary and some other medical sources, is a reasonable conclusion.

From an even more positivist angle, Grant then asks if this picture of slightly healthier women than men reflects a broader social reality. The slightly lower mortality rates for women than men from Harriet Zurndorfer's study of the Fan lineage in the same region support this point.[35] Less mobility probably sheltered elite women from the infectious diseases to which their more mobile merchant and official husbands would have more likely been exposed. These arguments are thought provoking, but from a demographic perspective unconvincing. Wang's female patients appeared to have been a highly select group comprised of mostly elite, many older, and otherwise relatively well-off women. These figures are not generally representative of the range of women in the Huizhou region during the mid-Ming dynasty. Except for the case of an elderly village woman in her fifties,[36] Wang did not see peasant women, concubines, or prostitutes in his clinic or in their homes, at least not as their physician. Even though he refers to the concubines of some of his depleted male patients, he never discusses the consequences of sexual indulgence on their health (pp. 122-24). The lives of these three types of women, however, would have been profoundly changed by the transformations in the Huizhou economy and these women possibly exposed to more serious illnesses than their elite female contemporaries. Yet, obviously, all were excluded from the social networks from which Wang Ji culled his female patients. The general impression that the *Stone Mountain* cases convey of slightly sicker male than female patients does not, however, reflect an actual social reality so much as it manifests the moral lens through which Wang filtered his social world and made meaning of his medical cases.[37]

Etiology

Because the most significant and interesting gender differences are found in Wang's discussions of etiology, I have chosen to discuss them last. Whereas he warned men about excessive sexual activity, he wrote about women being apprehensive or repressed about sex. Emotions were gendered as well in that more men suffered from disorders related to anger and anxiety, whereas women experienced problems stemming from pensiveness or sorrow. Emotional states tended to be cast as central in women and incidental in men. In

---

[35] Harriet T. Zurndorfer, *Change and Continuity in Chinese Local History: The Development of Hui-chou Prefecture 800-1800* (Leiden: Brill, 1989).

[36] *Shishan yi'an* (*juan* 2), in *Wang Shishan Yixue quanshu*, 81b.

[37] See the main distinction between social history and cultural history analysis that Fissell makes in "Making Meaning from the Margins," 366-67.

general, Wang blamed excessive sexual activity, alcohol, and rich food for most male disorders and attributed nonreproductive female illnesses to excessive or uncontrolled emotions.

The third fascicle contains a cluster of six disorders related to emotions that further support Grant's conclusions. The first four female cases following an essay on the *wu zhi* 五志 (the five emotions) were grouped together as examples of emotional counter-therapy, a practice of inciting specific emotions in a patient in order to right an imbalance according to the conquest cycle of the five phases.[38] Here men suffer from excessive joy (*xi* 喜) and anxiety (*you* 憂), women from pensiveness (*si* 思) and fright (*jing* 驚). Whereas in fiction as well as in medicine Chinese men more than women suffer from sexual overindulgence, women inordinately endure sexual repression and manifest bodily depletion.[39] Men actively contract syphilis in the brothels; women passively fall prey to seductive fox spirits or fantasies of illicit sex in their dreams. Men have too much sex; women possess excessive desire and repressed passion.[40]

Wang's view of depleted males may have been as much a response to perceived social ills, however, as an acknowledgement of compromised masculinity. Such males often appear as pale, weak, and fragile as female ghosts and sickly women—the two literary tropes of hyperfemininity.[41] From a more expanded gender perspective, Wang's preference for restoratives may have been implicitly as much about restoring the masculinity of his male patients as they were explicitly about treating their depletions. This implicit intention would align well with Furth's interpretation of Zhu Zhenheng's earlier doctrines of "Yang Surplus and Yin Deficiency" as aligning the medical body with neo-Confucian metaphysics and a new construction of literati masculinity.[42] Grant observes that Wang also recommends

---

[38] For an explanation of this form of therapy, see Sivin, "Emotional Counter-Therapy," 1-6.

[39] See especially the section "The Ghost's Body and Medical Images of Women," 244-52, in Judith T. Zeitlin, "Embodying the Disembodied: Representations of Ghosts and the Feminine," in Ellen Widmer and Kang-I Sun Chang, eds., *Writing Women in Late Imperial China* (Stanford: Stanford University Press, 1997), 242-63.

[40] See "The Experience of Venereal Disease in Ming and Qing China," in Andrew David Schonebaum, "Fictional Medicine: Diseases, Doctors and the Curative Properties of Chinese Fiction" (Ph.D. diss., Columbia University, 2004), 256-68.

[41] On the connections between hyperfemininity and masculinity, see Zeitlin, "Embodying the Disembodied," 244-48.

[42] See "The Body of Yang Surplus and Yin Deficiency," in Furth, *A Flourishing Yin*, 145-51.

self-cultivation only to his male patients, as an antidote to their over-indulgence in sex, alcohol, and diet. Women are neither susceptible to such excesses nor capable of moral self-cultivation (p. 134). This line of reasoning relates well with Grant's analysis of Wang's self-portrayal and biography of his father Wang Wei 汪渭 (1433-1515) as models of the moderate behaviors and moral values of the ideal Confucian male that his upwardly mobile but morally wayward male patients should emulate.

Final Assessment

Grant engages with women in Chinese medical history as a lawyer would approach a legal case. By using new evidence from the medical case histories of one sixteenth-century physician, she tests the universal applicability of previous scholars' generalizations about Chinese conceptions of women, which had been based on a broader reading of medical, literary, and official sources. Her emphasis on the exceptions to the rule that "Blood rules women" forces a revision of previous assessments. Her instincts to examine the fissures between abstract doctrine and concrete clinical practice are as sound as the method promises to be long lasting. Her approach to see how gender manifests in every stage of the clinical encounter is illuminating. Her insight, in other words, that differences between women (reproductive versus nonreproductive disorders) may have been even greater than differences between the sexes suggests a new dimension for further reflection. When Wang dispenses moral advice and self-cultivation along with replenishing herbs to his depleted male patients, we see how cultural and historical factors intersected with his medical diagnoses and therapeutic interventions. The connection made between Wang's dominant medical diagnosis of male depletion and his cultural perceptions of male decadence in the newly emergent Huizhou mercantile culture significantly contributes to the field. A stimulating yet ultimately tantalizing book, Grant's interpretation of the *Stone Mountain Medical Case Histories* leaves room for others to break new ground and reap richer harvests in the history of women and gender in Chinese medicine.

REVIEWS

ZHANG Zhibin 張志斌. *Gudai Zhongyi fuchanke jibingshi* 古代中醫婦產科疾病史 (A history of obstetrical and gynecological diseases in ancient China) Beijing: Zhongyi guzi chubanshe, 2000. 438 pp. RMB 22. ISBN 7-80013-923-9

Traditional Chinese medicine, once either consigned to the sphere of the mystical or simply underrated, now attracts much attention. Many people are impressed with its emphasis on seeking harmony between the processes of the universe and human activities, which seems to offer an alternative to those who feel threatened by the increasing intrusion of science into human life. It is hardly surprising, therefore, that the history of Chinese medicine has grown into an independent academic discipline, embracing such themes as the evolution of the philosophy of Chinese medicine, Chinese medical training and institutions past and present, the history of the Chinese medical profession, different types of diseases in ancient China, and the social and cultural factors affecting the practice of Chinese medicine. That the website http://www.albion.edu/history/chimed/scholar.html alone names more than 120 Asian and Western scholars who are conducting specialized research into the history of Chinese medicine testifies to the growing influence and popularity of this field of study.

In Zhang Zhibin's *Gudai Zhongyi fuchanke jibingshi* 古代中醫婦產科疾病史 (A history of obstetrical and gynecological diseases in ancient China), the introduction makes it clear that she is focusing on the causes, symptoms, diagnoses, prevention, and treatment of obstetrical and gynecological diseases as recorded in Chinese historical sources. Pediatric diseases, though closely related to these, are not central to her research (p. 5). Adopting a rather traditional approach, this book is concerned with how these issues were dealt with through history. Its four major chapters take us in chronological order from the earliest times, through the Han, Qin, Sui and Tang dynasties; the Song, Jin, and Yuan dynasties; and finally the Ming and Qing dynasties. For Zhang, although the oracles found in the Shang dynasty (1523 BCE -1027 BCE) already contained early findings about obstetrical and gynecological diseases, systematic studies of these maladies began only after supernatural elements were removed from the picture

Also available online – www.brill.nl

in Chinese medicine. Through trial and error, rationalization and intellectualization, scholars and medical researchers in the Han, Qin, Sui, and Tang dynasties gradually turned their observations and experiences into a system of knowledge in which the diseases related to menstruation, pregnancy, and postmaternal problems, as well as morbid leucorrhoea, were studied as specific subjects.

The study of obstetrical and gynecological diseases entered a new phase in the Song dynasty, in which ancient Chinese civilization reached one of its golden ages. Thanks to the emergence of empirical methods (p. 166) that challenged traditional values and behaviors, medical researchers and practitioners in this period examined these diseases in a much more scientific manner, creating not only voluminous pathological analyses of menstrual disorders, miscarriage, and other postmaternal diseases (pp 171-76), but also new precautions and treatments founded upon inductive reasoning (pp. 185-93). Zhang further points out that as a result of the advances in their knowledge of biology and psychology, medical researchers in the Ming and Qing dynasties became aware of the relationship between women's general health and mental conditions, and obstetrical and gynecological diseases (pp. 251-59). Their great work helped transform the study of obstetrical and gynecological diseases into a branch of the health sciences whose value should not be overlooked even today.

Zhang's book, which draws principally on primary sources, offers by far the most detailed and well-documented study on the subject to date, admitting us to the wisdom of ancient Chinese obstetricians and gynecologists. However, Zhang's penchant for adopting a philological approach leaves her little room to conceive traditional Chinese medicine as a cultural and social product, whose development was in many ways determined by exogenous as well as endogenous factors. It will perhaps not be superfluous here to recount very briefly the philosophical base upon which Chinese medicine is founded. Basically, traditional Chinese medicine perceives that the life cycle of human beings, like everything in the universe, is governed by a set of principles produced by the interactions of the two opposites (*yin* 陰 and *yang* 陽, or darkness and brightness, or female and male) and the five elements (metal, wood, water, fire, and earth). Compliance with these principles brings order and well-being. Any attempt to defy them leads to chaos and disorder. Sicknesses are thus disorders inside human bodies caused by activities which run counter to these principles.

Ancient Chinese understandings and treatments of obstetrical and gynecological diseases cannot be fully understood without reference to this correspondence theory, as it is sometimes called. Surprisingly, Zhang's book, in paying rather little attention to the influence of the correspondence theory, creates an impression that the study of obstetrical and gynecological diseases in ancient China had little to do with the philosophy of Chinese medicine. It is true that nowadays not all practitioners of Chinese medicine subscribe to the correspondence theory. Zhang, however, seems to have adopted the idea that obstetrical and gynecological diseases in pre-modern China can be understood outside the traditional philosophical framework, but without making enough effort to establish or justify this position.

One major contribution of gender studies since the 1960s has been the dissemination of the view that manhood as well as womanhood is socially and culturally constructed rather than biologically determined. Women are not necessarily willing mothers or obedient wives. They are not submissive or sexually inactive by virtue of their nature as women. Their characteristics are rather a result of socialization and the influence of mainstream culture. Women's studies on one hand provide us with new perspectives for reconsidering the social and biological needs and conditions of women, and on the other, awaken us to an awareness of the unreasonableness of practices and institutions developing out of our misconceptions of women. As Thomas Kuhn pointed out in his masterpiece, *The Structure of Scientific Revolution*, published over thirty years ago, social, cultural, and institutional factors such as beliefs, the consensus shared by scientists, and the norms created by scientific communities shape scientific research more than intellectual factors do. The patrimonial values that have hitherto dominated human societies, and the social practices and institutions stemming from these values, probably dictate the understanding of women's bodies and health that doctors and medical experts construct. The relationship between gender and the inquiry into obstetrical and gynecological diseases, since they affect women exclusively, remains an interesting question that Zhang and other historians of Chinese medicine need to address.

Zhang's book aims to show the achievements in the study of obstetrical and gynecological diseases in China in the last three millennia. It is perhaps too ambitious a project. China's culture and society, as well as the state of its science and technology, have undergone great changes in the course of its long history, many of them closely related to the development of medical studies. For example, urbanization since the Song dynasty, the movement of the Chinese population from inland to coastal areas, ecological and climatic changes that have affected Chinese people's habits and lifestyles, growing contact with the West, the encounter between Chinese medicine and modern Western science—all these exerted direct and indirect influences on the theory and practice of Chinese medicine, including the study of obstetrical and gynecological diseases. These subjects are too complex to be dealt with in a single volume.

Ricardo King-sang Mak
Hong Kong Baptist University

BIBLIOGRAPHY OF SECONDARY SOURCES ON MEDICINE AND GENDER: EARLY IMPERIAL CHINA

BY

CHARLOTTE FURTH
(University of Southern California)

Note: The bibliography here is necessarily selective, building on a few classic and recent secondary sources important to the authors of the essays in this special issue of Nan Nü. *Given that the intersection of medicine and gender history draws upon a large volume of works on both topics, I have chosen to emphasize sources on medicine. Similarly, I have stressed the early empire (Han through Song dynasties) which is less well studied than the late imperial era. My thanks to Angela Leung for her suggestions and additions to this list.*

Ahern, Emily M. "The Power and Pollution of Chinese Women," in Margery Wolf and Roxane Witke, eds., *Women in Chinese Society* (Stanford: Stanford University Press, 1975), pp. 193-214.

Anonymous. *Zhongguo yiyao shihua*, 中国医药史话 (Historical anecdotes on Chinese medicine) (Taibei: Mingwen shuju, 1983).

Bray, Francesca. "A Deathly Disorder: Understanding Women's Health in Late Imperial China." in Don Bates, ed., *Knowledge and the Scholarly Medical Traditions* (Cambridge, England: Cambridge University Press, 1995), pp. 235-50.

—— *Technology and Gender: Fabrics of Power in Late Imperial China* (Berkeley, California: University of California Press, 1995).

Cahill, Suzanne E. *Women and the Dao : Records of the Transcendents of the Fortified Walled City of Du Guangting (850-933)* (Cambridge, Mass: Three Pine Press [forthcoming, 2006]).

Cass, Victoria. "Female Healers in the Ming and the Lodge of Ritual and Ceremony," *Journal of the American Oriental Society* 106.1 (1986):233-40.

Chen Hsiu-fen. "Wind Malady as Madness in Medieval China: Some Threads from the Dunhuang Medical Manuscript," in Vivienne Lo and Christopher Cullen, eds., *Medieval Chinese Medicine: The Dunhuang Medical Manuscripts* (London and New York: Routledge Curzon, 2005), pp. 345-362.

Cole, Alan. *Mothers and Sons in Chinese Buddhism* (Stanford, California: Stanford University Press, 1998).

Cooper, William and Nathan Sivin. "Man as a Medicine: Pharmacological and Ritual Aspects of Traditional Therapy Using Drugs Derived from the Human Body," in Nakayama Shigeru and Nathan Sivin, eds., *Chinese Science: Explorations of an Ancient Tradition* (Cambridge, Mass.: MIT Press, 1973), pp. 203-272.

Cullen, Christopher. "Patients and Healers in Late Imperial China: Evidence from the *Jinpingmei*," *History of Science* 31(1993): 99-150.

Also available online – www.brill.nl

Despeux, Catherine. *Immortelles de la Chine ancienne: Taoism et alchemie feminine.* (Paris: Pardes, 1990).
—— "The System of Five Circulatory Phases and Six Seasonal Influences (Wuyun Liuqi), a Source of Innovation in Medicine under the Song (960-1279)," in Elisabeth Hsu, ed., *Innovation in Chinese Medicine,* (Cambridge: Cambridge University Press, 2001), pp. 121-166.
—— (Penelope Barrett, trans.), "Visual Representations of the Body in Chinese Medical and Daoist Texts from the Song to the Qing Period," *Asian Medicine: Tradition and Modernity* 1 (2005): 10-50.
Despeux, Catherine and Frédéric Obringer. eds., *La maladie dans la Chine médiévale: la toux* (Paris: Editions L'Harmattan, 1997).
DeWoskin, Kenneth J. *Doctors, Diviners and Magicians of Ancient China: Biographies of Fang-shih* (New York: Columbia University Press, 1983).
Ding Guangdi 丁光迪. *Jin Yuan yixue pingxi* 金元医学评析 (Analysis of medical learning of the Jin and Yuan periods) (Beijing: Renmin weisheng chubanshe, 1999).
Ebrey, Patricia. *The Inner Quarters: Marriage and the Lives of Chinese Women in the Song Period* (Berkeley: University of California Press, 1993).
Engelhardt, Ute. "Dietetics in Tang China and the First Extant Works of Materia Dietetica," in Elisabeth Hsu, ed., *Innovation in Chinese Medicine* (Cambridge: Cambridge University Press, 2001), pp. 173-191.
Fan Xingzhun 范行准. *Zhongguo yixue shilüe* 中国医学史略 (Brief history of Chinese medicine) (Beijing: Zhongyi guji chubanshe, 1986).
——. *Zhongguo bingshi xinyi* 中国病史新义 (Beijing: Zhongguo guji chubanshe, 1989).
Fu Weikang 傅维康 et al. *Zhongguo yixue shi* 中国医学史 (History of China's medical learning) (Shanghai: Zhongyi xueyuan chubanshe, 1990).
Furth, Charlotte. "Concepts of Pregnancy, Childbirth and Infancy in Ch'ing Dynasty China," *Journal of Asian Studies* 46.1 (1987): 17-35.
—— "Rethinking Van Gulik: Sexuality and Reproduction in Traditional Chinese Medicine," in Christina K. Gilmartin, Gail Hershatter, et al., eds., *Engendering China: Women, Culture and the State.* (Cambridge, Mass: Harvard University Press, 1994), pp. 125-46.
—— "From Birth to Birth: The Growing Body in Chinese Medicine," in Anne Behnke Kinney, ed., *Chinese Views of Childhood* (Honolulu: University of Hawai'i Press, 1995), pp. 157-91.
—— *A Flourishing Yin: Gender in China's Medical History 960-1665* (Berkeley: University of California Press, 1999) .
Ge Jianmin 盖建民. *Daojiao Yixue* 道教医学 (Daoist medical learning) (Beijing: Zongjiao wenhua chubanshe, 1999).
Goldin, Paul R. *The Culture of Sex in Ancient China* (Honolulu: University of Hawaii Press, 2002).
Goldschmidt, Asaf. "The Transformations of Chinese Medicine During the Northern Song Dynasty (AD 960-1127)," Ph.D. diss., University of Pennsylvania, 1999.
—— "Changing Standards: Tracing Changes in Acu-moxa Therapy during the Transition from the Tang to the Song Dynasties," *East Asian Science, Technology and Medicine* 18 (2001):75-111.
—— "The Song Discontinuity: Rapid Innovation in Northern Song Dynasty Medicine," *Asian Medicine: Tradition and Modernity* 1 (2005): 52-90.
Guo Licheng 郭立诚. *Zhongguo shengyu lisu kao* 中国生育礼俗考 (Investigation of Chinese childbirth rituals and customs) (Taipei: Wenshezhe chubanshe, 1971).
Grant, Beata. "The Spiritual Saga of Woman Huang: From Pollution to Purification,"

in David Johnson, ed., *Ritual Operatic Ritual: Mu-lien Rescues His Mother in Chinese Popular Culture* (Berkeley: Institute of East Asian Studies, 1989), pp. 224-231.

Grant, Joanna. *A Chinese Physician: Wang Ji and the Stone Mountain Medical Case Histories* (London: Routledge Curzon 2003).

Harper, Donald. *Early Chinese Medical Literature: the Mawangdui Medical Manuscripts* (London & New York: Kegan Paul International, 1998).

—— "Iatromancy, Diagnosis and Prognosis in Early Chinese Medicine," in Elisabeth Hsu, ed., *Innovation in Chinese Medicine* (Cambridge: Cambridge University Press, 2001), pp. 99-120.

—— "Ancient and Medieval Chinese Recipes for Aphrodisiacs and Philters," *Asian Medicine:Tradition and Modernity* 1 (2005): 91-100.

He Shixi 何时希. *Zhenben nüke yishu ji yi bazhong* 珍本女科医书辑佚八种 (A precious compilation of eight lost medical books on female disorders) (Shanghai: Xuelin chubanshe, 1984).

Hinrichs, T. J. "The Medical Transforming of Governance and Southern Customs in Song Dynasty China (960-1279 CE)," Ph.D. diss., Harvard University, 2004.

Hsiung Ping-chen (Xiong Bingzhen 熊秉真). *You you: chuantong Zhongguo de qiangbao zhi dao* 幼幼: 传统中国的襁褓之道 (The way of caring for the newborn in traditional China) (Taipei: Lianjing chuban shiye gongsi, 1995).

—— "To Nurse the Young: Breastfeeding and Infant Feeding in Late Imperial China," *Journal of Family History* 20.3 (1995): 217-238.

—— *Tender Voyage: Children and Childhood in Late Imperial China* (Stanford, California: Stanford University Press, 2005).

—— "Recipes of Planting the Seeds and Songs of Sleeping Alone: A Profile of Male Body Culture in Ming-Ch'ing China," *Late Imperial China* 26.2 (December 2005) [forthcoming].

Hsü Cho-yun 许倬云. "Handai jiating daxiao" 汉代家庭大小 (All about Han dynasty households), in Hsü Cho-yun, ed. *Qiongqubian* 求古编 (Seeking antiquity collection) (Taipei: Lianjing chubanshe, 1982).

Hsu, Elisabeth. "Pulse Diagnostics in the Western Han: How Mai and Qi Determine Bing," in Elisabeth Hsu, ed., *Innovation in Chinese Medicine* (Cambridge: Cambridge University Press, 2001), pp. 51-91.

——. ed., *Innovation in Chinese Medicine* (Cambridge: Cambridge University Press, 2001).

Kinney, Anne Behnke. "Infant Abandonment in Early China," *Early China* 18 (1993): 107-38.

——, ed. *Chinese Views of Childhood* (University of Hawai'i Press, 1995).

Kuriyama, Shigehisa. "The Imagination of Winds and the Development of the Chinese Conception of the Body," in Angela Zito and Tani E. Barlow, eds., *Body, Subject and Power in China.* (Chicago: University of Chicago Press, 1994), pp. 23-41.

—— *The Expressiveness of the Body and the Divergence of Greek and Chinese Medicine* (New York: Zone Books, 1999).

—— "Visual Knowledge in Classical Chinese Medicine," in Don Bates, ed., *Knowledge and the Scholarly Medical Traditions* (Cambridge: Cambridge University Press, 1995), pp. 205-234.

——. "Angry Women and the History of Chinese Medicine," in Michael Worton and Nana Wilson-Tagoe, eds., *National Healths: Gender, Sexuality and Health in a Cross-Cultural Context* (London: UCL press, 2004), pp 179-190.

Ko, Dorothy. "The Body as Attire: the Shifting Meanings of Foot-binding in seventeenth-century China," *Journal of Women's History,* 8 (1997). 8-27.

—— *Every Step a Lotus, Shoes for Bound Feet* (Berkeley: University of California Press, 2001).

—— *Cinderella's Sisters: A Revisionist History of Footbinding* (Berkeley: University of California Press 2005).
Lee Jender (Li Zhende 李贞德). "Han-Sui zhijian di shengzi buju wenti," 汉隋之间的生子不举问题 (The problem of infanticide in late antiquity and early medieval China), *Bulletin of the Institute of History and Philology, Academia Sinica* 中央研究院历史语言研究所集刊 66.3 (1995): 747-812.
—— "Han-Tang zhijian yishu zhong de shengchan zhi dao" 汉唐之间医术中的生产之道 (Childbirth in the medical writings of late antiquity and early medieval China), *Bulletin of the Institute of History and Philology, Academia Sinica*, 67.3 (1996): 533-654.
—— "Han-Tang zhijian qiuzi yifang shitan—ianluan fuke lanshang yu xingbie lunshu" 汉唐之间求子医方试探—兼论妇科滥觞与性别论述 (Reproductive medicine in late antiquity and early medieval China—gender discourse and the birth of gynecology), *Bulletin of the Institute of History and Philology, Academia Sinica* 68.2 (1997):283-367.
—— "Han-Tang zhijian di nüxing yiliao zhaogu zhe" 汉唐之间的女性医疗照顾者 (The medical care of women in late antiquity and early medieval China), *Taida lishi xuebao* 台大历史学报 23 (1999): 123-156.
—— "Han-Wei Liuchao di rumu" 汉魏六朝的乳母 (Wet nurses in the Han, Wei and Six Dynasties period), *Bulletin of the Institute of History and Philology, Academia Sinica* 70.2 (1999): 439-481.
—— "Wet Nurses in Early Imperial China" *Nan Nü* 2.1(2000) 1-39.
—— "Han-Tang zhijian jiating zhong de jiankang zhaogu yu xingbie" 汉唐之间家庭中的健康照顾与性别 (Gender and family health care in late antiquity and early medieval China), in Huang Kewu 黃克武, ed., *Di san jie guoji hanxue huiyi lunwenji: xingbie yu yiliao* 第三届国际汉学会议论文集：性别与医疗 (Gender and medicine: papers from the third international conference on Sinology), Institute of Modern History, Academia Sinica 中央研究院近代史研究所 (2001), pp. 1-50.
—— "Han-Tang zhijian yifang zhong di jijian furen yu nüti wei yao" 汉唐之间医方中的忌见妇人与女体为药 (Female body as medicine and medicinal taboos surrounding women in late antiquity and early medieval China), *Xin shixue*新史学 13.4 (2002): 1-36.
—— "Tangdai di xingbie yu yiliao" 唐代的性别与医疗 (Gender and medicine in Tang dynasty China), in Deng Xiaonan 邓小南, ed., *Tang-Song nüxing yu shehui* 唐宋女性与社会 (Women and society in the Tang and Song dynasties) (Shanghai: Cishu chubanshe, 2003).
—— "'*Ishinpo*' lun 'furen zhubing suoyou' jiqi xiangguan wenti" "医心方"论"妇人诸病所由"及其相关问题 ('Ishinpo' discussion of 'The origins of women's disorders' and related questions), *Tsing Hua Journal of Chinese Studies* 清华学报 34.2 (2004): 479-511.
—— "Xiaoji kao—jian lun Zhongguo guyi zhe dui xile de taidu" 笑疾考—兼論中國中古醫者對喜樂的態度 ('Laughing disorders' and the medical discourse of joy in early imperial China), *Bulletin of the Institute of History and Philology, Academia Sinica* 75.1 (2004): 99-148.
—— "Gender and Medicine in Tang China," *Asia Major* 16.2 (2003): 1-32.
Leung Ki Che, Angela (Liang Qizi 梁其姿). "Women Practicing Medicine in Premodern China," in Harriet T. Zurndorfer, ed., *Chinese Women in the Imperial Past: New Perspectives* (Leiden: Brill, 1999), pp. 101-34.
—— "Zhongguo mafeng bing gainian yanbian di lishi" 中國痲風病概念演變的歷史 (The historical nosology of 'li/lai' [leprosy] in China), *Bulletin of the Institute of History and Philology, Academia Sinica* 70.2 (1999): 399-438.
—— "Jibing yu fangtu zhi guanxi:Yuan zhi Ming Qing jian yi jie de kanfa "疾病与方土之关系:元至明清间医界的看法 (The relationship of disease and environment:

attitudes in medical circles from Yuan to Ming-Qing times), Huang Kewu, ed., *Di san jie guoji hanxue huiyi lunwenji: xingbie yu yiliao* 第三届国际汉学会议论文集：性别与医疗 (Papers from the Third international conference on Sinology), Institute of Modern History, Academia Sinica 中央研究院近代史研究所 (2001), pp. 165-212.

—— "Medical Learning from the Song to the Ming," in Paul Jakov Smith and Richard von Glahn, eds., *The Song-Yuan-Ming Transition in Chinese History* (Cambridge, MA.: Harvard Asia Center 2003), pp. 374-400.

Li Bozhong 李伯重. "Duotai, biyun yu jueyu—Song-Yuan-Ming-Qing Jiang-Zhe diqu di jieyu fangfa ji qi yunyong yu chuanbo" 堕胎、避孕与绝育—宋元明清时期江浙地区的节育方法及其运用与传播 (Abortion, contraception and sterilization—The use and transmission of birth control methods in Jiangnan in the Song, Yuan Ming and Qing periods), *Zhongguo xueshu* 中国学术 1(2000): 71-99.

Li Jianmin 李建民. "Mawangdui Hanmu boshu 'yuzang maibo tu' jianzheng" 马王堆汉墓帛书禹藏埋胞图笺证 (Textual evidence relating to the "Storehouse of Yu placenta burial chart" from the Mawangdui tomb manscripts), *Bulletin of the Institute of History and Philology, Academia Sinica* 65.4 (1994): 725-832.

—— "Furen meidao kao: chuantong jiating di chongtu yu huajie fangshu" "妇人媚道"考—传统家庭的冲突与化解方术 (Study of "The woman's way of charming"—traditional family conflicts and techniques of resolution), *Xin shixue* 新史学 7.4 (1996): 1-32.

—— "Wang Mang yu Wangsun Qing: ji gongyuan yi shiji de renti kubo shiyan" 王莽与王孙庆—记公元一世紀的人体刳剥实验 (Wang Mang and Wangsun Qing: records of the practice of human dissection in the first century CE), *Xin shixue* 新史学 10.4(1999): 1-30.

—— "Dumai yu Zhongguo zaoqi yangsheng shijian: qi jing ba mai di xin yanjiu zhi er" 督脉与中国早期养生实践：奇经八脉的新研究之二 (The superintendent channel and the practice of nourishing life in early China: new research on the eight odd channel pulses, number two), *Bulletin of the Institute of History and Philology Academia Sinica* 76.2 (2005):249-314.

Li Jingwei 李经纬. "Bei Song huangdi yu yixue" 北宋皇帝与医学 (Northern Song emperors and medicine), *Zhongguo keji shiliao* 中国科技史料 10.3(1990): 3-20.

Li Jingwei 李经纬 and Li Zhidong 李志东. *Zhongguo gudai yixue shilue*中国古代医学史略 (Outline history of China's ancient medical learning) (Shijiazhuang: Heibei kexue jishu chubanshe, 1990).

Li Tao (Lee T'ao 李濤). "A Brief History of Obstetrics and Gynecology in China from Ancient Times to Before the Opium War," *Chinese Medical Journal* 77 (1958): 477-86.

Li Yinhe 李银河. *Shengyu yu Zhongguo cunluo wenhua* 生育与中国村落文化 (Childbirth and China's village culture) (Hong Kong: Oxford University Press, 1993).

Li Yuzhen 李玉珍. "Fojiao piyu wenxue zhong de nannü meise yu qingyu: zhuiqiu meili de zongjiao hanyi" 佛教譬喻文学中的男女美色与情欲：追求美丽的宗教意涵 (Sex and desire in Buddhist Avadana literature: seeking the hidden religious meaning of beauty), *Xin shixue* 新史学 10.4 (1999): 31-66.

Liang Jun 梁峻. *Zhongguo gudai yizheng shilüe* 中国古代医政史略 (Brief history of medicine and the state in ancient China) (Urumqi: Nei Menggu renmin chubanshe, 1995).

Liao Yuqun 廖育群. "Chen Yanzhi yu '*Xiaopinfang*' yanjiu de xin jinzhan" 陈延之与小品方研究的新进展 (Chen Yanzhi and new developments in research on '*Xiaopinfang*'), *Zhonghua yishi zazhi* 中华医史杂志 17.2 (1987): 74-75.

Liu Jingzhen 刘静贞. "Cong sun zi huai tai di baoying chuanshuo kan Song dai funü di shengyu wenti" 从损子坏胎的报应传说看宋代妇女的生育问题 (The question of childbearing in the Song dynasty from the perspective of tales of retribution from aborted fetuses and dead infants), *Dalu zazhi* 大陆杂志 90.1 (1995): 25-38.

Liu Lexian. "Love Charms Among the Dunhuang Manuscripts," in Vivienne Lo and Christopher Cullen, eds., *Medieval Chinese Medicine: The Dunhuang Medical Manuscripts* (London and New York: Routledge Curzon, 2005), pp. 165-75.

Liu Zenggui 劉增貴. "Handai hunyin zhidu" 汉代婚姻制度 (The institution of marriage in the Han dynasty) (Taipei: Huashi chubanshe, 1982).

Lo, Vivienne. "Crossing the *neiguan* 內關 "Inner Pass": A *nei/wai* 内外 "Inner/Outer" Distinction in Early Chinese Medicine," *East Asian Science, Technology and Medicine* 17(2000): 15-65.

—— "The Influence of Nurturing Life Culture on the Development of Western Han Acumoxa Therapy," in Elisabeth Hsu, ed., *Innovation in Chinese Medicine* (Cambridge: Cambridge University Press, 2001), pp.19-50.

—— and Christopher Cullen, eds., *Medieval Chinese Medicine: The Dunhuang Medical Manuscripts* (London and New York: Routledge Curzon 2005).

—— "Quick and Easy Chinese Medicine: the Dunhuang Moxibustian Charts," in Vivienne Lo and Christopher Cullen, eds., *Medieval Chinese Medicine; the Dunhuang Medical Manuscripts* (London and New York: Routledge Curzon 2005), pp. 227-51.

Luo Yuankai 罗元恺., ed., *Zhongyi fuke xue* 中医妇科学 (The study of medicine for women in Chinese medicine) (Taipei: Zhiyin chubanshe, 1997).

Ma Dazheng 马大正. *Zhongguo fuchanke fazhan shi* 中国妇产科发展史 (A history of the development of gynecology and obstetrics in China) (Xi'an: Shanxi kexue jiaoyu chubanshe, 1991).

Ma Jixing马继兴. "Taichanshu kaoshi" 胎产书考释 (Annotated text of the 'book of pregnancy and birth') in *Mawangdui guyishu kaoshi* 马王堆古医书考释 (Study and interpretation of the ancient medical manuscripts from Mawangdui) (Changsha: Hunan kexue jishu chubanshe, 1992).

Needham, Joseph, with the collaboration of Lu Gwei-Djen. *Science and Civilization in China. Vol 5. Chemistry and Chemical Technology. Part 5. Spagyrical Discovery and Invention: Physiological Alchemy* (Cambridge: Cambridge University Press 1982).

——, with an introduction by Nathan Sivin. *Science and Civilization in China. Volume 6: Biology and Biological Technology. Part IV: Medicine* (Cambridge: Cambridge University Press, 2000)

Obringer, Frédéric. "A Song Innovation in Pharmacotherapy: Some Remarks on the Use of White Arsenic and Flowers of Arsenic," in Elisabeth Hsu, ed., *Innovation in Chinese Medicine* (Cambridge: Cambridge University Press, 2001), pp. 192-213.

—— *L'aconite et l'orpiment: drogues et poisons en Chine ancienne et médiévale* (Paris: Fayard, 1997).

Pu Muzhou 蒲慕洲.. "Shuihudi Qinjian rishu de shijie" 睡虎地秦简日书的世界 (The world of the Qin dynasty almanacs [in bamboo strips] from Shuihudi), *Bulletin of the Institute of History and Philosophy, Academia Sinica* 中央研究院历史研究所集刊 62.4 (1993): 623-75.

Qiu Zhonglin 邱仲麟. "Renyao yu xueqi: 'gegu' liaoqin xianxiang zhong de yiliao guannian" 人药与血气——"割股"疗亲现象中的医疗观念 (The human body as medicine and the vitalities of blood/qi—medical ideas about the phenomenon of "flesh cutting" to cure parents), *Xin shixue* 新史学 10.4(1999): 67-116.

Raphals, Lisa. "The Treatment of Women in a Second-century Medical Casebook," *Chinese Science*, 15 (1998): 7-28.

—— *Sharing the Light: Representations of Women and Virtue in Early China* (Albany: State University of New York Press, 1998).

Ren Yingqiu 任应秋. *Zhongyi gejia xueshuo* 中医各家学说 (Study of the schools of thought in Chinese medicine) (Shanghai: Kexue zhishu chubanshe, 1980).

Rouzer, Paul. *Articulated Ladies: Gender and the Male community in Early Chinese Texts.* (Harvard East Asia Center, 2001).

Sivin, Nathan. "State, Cosmos and the Body in the Last Three Centuries B.C.," *Harvard Journal of Asiatic Studies* 55.1(1995): 5-37.

—— "Text and Experience in Classical Chinese Medicine," in Don Bates ed., *Knowledge and the Scholarly Medical Traditions* (Cambridge: Cambridge University Press, 1995).

—— "Emotional Counter-therapy," in Nathan Sivin, *Medicine, Philosophy and Religion in Ancient China: Researches and Reflections* (Aldershot, Hants: Variorum 1995) pp. 1-19.

Song Shugong 宋书功. *Zhongguo gudai fangshi yangsheng jiyao* 中国古代房室养生集要 (Essentials on nourishing life in the bed-chamber in ancient China) (Beijing: Xinhua shudian, 1991).

Strickmann, Michel. *Chinese Magical Medicine.* (Stanford: Stanford University Press 2002).

Sumiyo Umekawa. "*Tiandi yinyang jiaohuang dalefu* and the Art of the Bedchamber" in Vivienne Lo and Christopher Cullen, eds., *Medieval Chinese Medicine: The Dunhuang Medical Manuscripts* (London and New York: Routledge Curzon 2005), pp. 252-77.

Tu Chengsheng 杜正胜 (Du Zhengsheng). "Lizhi, jiazu yu lunli" 理智, 家族与伦理 (Reason, family and ethics) in Tu Chengsheng, ed., *Gudai shehui yu guojia* 古代社会与国家 (Ancient society and nation) (Taipei: Yunchen wenhua chubanshe, 1992).

Unschuld, Paul U. *Medical Ethics in Imperial China: A Study in Historical Anthropology.* (Berkeley: University of California, Press, 1979).

—— *Medicine in China: a History of Ideas* (Berkeley: University of California Press, 1985).

—— *Medicine in China: Historical Artifacts and Images.* (Munich-London-New York: Prestel, 2000).

Valussi, Elena. "Beheading the Red Dragon: a History of Female Inner Alchemy in Late Imperial China," Ph.D. diss., SOAS, University of London, 2003.

Van Gulik, R. H. *Sexual Life in Ancient China.* (Leiden: E. J, Brill, 1974; reprinted in 2003 with an introduction by Paul R. Goldin).

Wang, Robin. ed. *Images of Women in Chinese Thought and Culture* (Indiana and Cambridge: Hackett Publishing Company, 2003).

Wile, Douglas. *Art of the Bedchamber: the Chinese Sexual Yoga Classics Including Women's Solo Meditation Texts* (Albany, New York: State University of New York Press, 1992).

Wilms, Sabine. "The Female Body in Medieval China." Ph.D. diss., University of Arizona, 2002.

——. "The Transmission of Medical Knowledge on 'Nuturing the Fetus' in Ancient China," *Asian Medicine: Tradition and Modernity* 2 (2005): 1-39.

Wiseman, Nigel and Feng Ye, eds., *A Practical Dictionary of Chinese Medicine* (Brookline, MA: Paradigm Publications ,1998).

Wu Baoqi 吴宝琪.. "Song dai chanyu zhi fengsu yanjiu" 宋代产育之风俗研究 (Research on Song dynasty childbirth customs), *Henan daxue xuebao* 河南大学学报 1(1989): 39-45.

Wu Hung and Katherine R. Tsiang, eds. *Body and Face in Chinese Visual Culture* (Cambridge, Mass.: Harvard Asia Center, 2005).

Wu Yili. "Transmitted Secrets: the Doctors of the Lower Yangzi Region and Popular Gynecology in Late Imperial China," Ph.D. diss., Yale University, 2000.

____ "The Bamboo Grove Monastery and Popular Gynecology in Qing China," *Late Imperial China* 21.1 (2000): 41-76.

____ "Ghost Fetuses, False Pregnancies, and the Parameters of Medical Uncertainty in Classical Chinese Gynecology," *Nan Nü* 4.2 (2002): 170-206.

Xie Liheng 谢利恒. *Zhongguo yixue yuanliu lun* 中国医学源流论 (On the evolution of Chinese medical learning) (Taibei: Guting shudian, 1970)

Yao Ping 姚平. *Tangdai funü di shengming licheng* 唐代妇女的生命历程 (The life cycle of Tang dynasty women) (Shanghai: Shanghai Guji chubanshe, 2004)

Yates, Robin. "Purity and Pollution in Early China," in Tsang Cheng-hwa 臧振華, ed. *Zhongguo kaoguxue yu lishixue zhi zhenghe guanxi* 中国考古学与历史学之整合貫系 (The complementary relationship of Chinese historical and archeological learning) (Taipei: Zhongyang yanjiuyuan lishi yuyan yanjiusuo, 1997), pp. 479-536.

Yu Chunfang. " A Sutra Promoting the White-robed Guanyin as a Giver of Sons," in Donald S. Lopez, ed., *Religions of China in Practice* (Princeton: Princeton University Press 1996), pp 97-105.

Yu Chunfang. *Kuan-yin: the Chinese Transformation of Avalokitesvara* (New York: Columbia University Press 2001).

Zhang Qiwen 张奇文, ed. *Fuke zabing* 妇科杂病 (Miscellaneous disorders of gynecology) (Beijing: Renmin weisheng chubanshe, 1995).

Zhang Zhibin 张志斌. *Gudai Zhongyi fuchanke jibing shi* 古代中医妇产科疾病史 (The history of women's diseases in ancient Chinese medicine) (Beijing: Zhongyi guji chubanshe, 2000).

Zhao Pushan 趙璞珊. *Zhongguo gudai yixue* 中国古代医学 (Medical learning of ancient China) (Beijing: Zhonghua shuju, 1983; reprinted in 1997).

Zheng Jinsheng 郑金生. "Mingdai nüyi Tan Yunxian ji qi yi'an 'Nüyi zayan'" 明代女医谈允贤及其医案"女医杂言" (Tan Yunxian, female physician of the Ming dynasty and her 'Sayings of a woman doctor'), *Zhonghua yishi zazhi* 中华医史杂志 29.3 (1999): 153-156.

—— "Riben neige wenku suo cang Yuan Ming yiji de chubu kaocha" 日本内阁文库所藏元明医籍的初步考察 (Preliminary investigation of Yuan and Ming medical texts stored in the Japanese imperial cabinet archive), in Huang Kewu, ed., *Di san jie guoji hanxue huiyi lunwenji: xingbie yu yiliao*, 213-41.

Zheng Yaru 郑雅如. "Qinggan yu zhidu: Wei Jin shiqi de muzi guanxi" 情感与制度：魏晋时期的母子关系 (Emotion and order: Wei and Jin era mother child relations), *Wenshi congkan series* 文史从刊 (Taipei: College of Liberal Arts, National Taiwan University, 2001).

INDEX

Nan Nü

Men, Women and Gender in China

Managing editor: Harriet T. ZURNDORFER

ISSN 1387-6805

Reprints of thematic issues

1. Paul S. ROPP, Paola ZAMPERINI and Harriet T. ZURNDORFER (eds.), *Passionate Women.* Female Suicide in Late Imperial China. 2001. ISBN 90 04 12018 1
2. Grace S. FONG, Nanxiu QIAN, Harriet T. ZURNDORFER (eds.), *Beyond Tradition and Modernity.* Gender, Genre, and Cosmopolitanism in Late Qing China. With an introduction by Susan L. MANN. 2004. ISBN 90 04 13894 3
3. Angela Ki Che LEUNG (ed.), *Medicine for Women in Imperial China.* 2006. ISBN 90 04 15196 6